Knowledge to Care
A Handbook for Care Assistants

Other books of interest:

The Royal Marsden Hospital Manual of Clinical Nursing Procedures
Third Edition
Edited by A. Phylip Pritchard and Jane Mallett
0–632–03387–8

The Royal Marsden Hospital Manual of Standards of Care
Edited by Joanna M. Luthert and Lorrain Robinson
0–632–03386–X

Health Promotion: Concepts and Practice
Edited by Alison Dines and Alan Cribb
0–632–03543–9

Sociology of Health and Health Care: An Introduction for Nurses
Steve Taylor and David Field
0–632–03402–5

Safer Lifting for Patient Care
Third Edition
M. Hollis
0–632–02892–0

Knowledge to Care
A Handbook for Care Assistants

Edited by

Christine A. McMahon
TD, RGN, RCNT, RNT, BSc

and

Joan Harding
BA, RGN, RM, RNT

b
Blackwell
Science

© 1994 Christine A. McMahon &
Joan Harding

Blackwell Science Ltd
Editorial Offices:
Osney Mead, Oxford OX2 0EL
25 John Street, London WC1 2BL
23 Ainslie Place, Edinburgh EH3 6AJ
238 Main Street, Cambridge
  Massachusetts 02142, USA
54 University Street, Carlton
  Victoria 3053, Australia

Other Editorial Offices:
Arnette Blackwell SA
  1, rue de Lille, 75007 Paris
  France

Blackwell Wissenschafts-Verlag GmbH
  Kurfürstendamm 57
  10707 Berlin
  Germany

  Feldgasse 13, A-1238 Wien
  Austria

First published 1993
Reprinted 1995, 1996

Set by DP Photosetting, Aylesbury, Bucks
Printed and bound in Great Britain
at the University Press, Cambridge

DISTRIBUTORS
Marston Book Services Ltd
PO Box 87
Oxford OX2 0DT
(*Orders*: Tel: 01865 791155
       Fax: 01865 791927
       Telex: 837515)

North America
Blackwell Science, Inc.
238 Main Street
Cambridge, MA 02142
(*Orders*: Tel: 800 215-1000
       617 876-7000
       Fax: 617 492-5263)

Australia
Blackwell Science Pty Ltd
54 University Street
Carlton, Victoria 3053
(*Orders*: Tel: 03 347-0300
       Fax: 03 349–3016)

A catalogue record for this book is available
from the British Library

ISBN 0–632–03585–4

Library of Congress
Cataloging in Publication Data

Knowledge to care: a handbook for care
assistants/edited by Christine A.
McMahon and Joan Harding.
    p.   cm.
    Includes bibliographical references and
index.
    ISBN 0–632–03585–4
    1. Nurses' aides.   2. Care of the sick.
I. McMahon, Christine A. II. Harding, Joan.
RT84.K57   1993
610.73'069'8–dc20   93-2082
                                        CIP

Contents

List of Contributors

Elizabeth Atchison, *MSc, RGN, RNT, Cert Ed*, Senior Lecturer (Macmillan), School of Acute Care, University of Luton, Luton and Dunstable Hospital, Luton.

Caroline Coleman, *RNMH, Cert in Adult and Further Education*, Staff Training and Development, Horizon NHS Trust, Trust HQ, Harperbury Hospital, Radlett.

Christine Cooper, *RGN, RM, CT Cert, Cert Ed*, Course Director, HCSW Training, St Bartholomew's College of Nursing and Midwifery, London.

Katie Cullinan, MSc, *Reg MCSLT*, Specialist Speech & Language Therapist, Home Choice, Finsbury Health Centre, London.

Joan Harding, *BA, RGN, RM. RNT*, former Project Officer, Barnet College of Nursing and Midwifery, Barnet.

Rita Gale, *City & Guilds 9292 (Staff Assessors Award), 9293 (Direct Training & Assessors Award), 7281/12 (Vocational Assessors Award)*, Assistant Patient Services Manager, The Middlesex/University College Hospitals, London.

Francis Guilfoyle, *RGN, RNT, Dip Educ, Dip Hum Sex*, former Lecturer in Human Sexuality, Sex and Relationship Therapist, Bloomsbury College of Nursing Education and Midwifery, London.

Christine McMahon, *TD, RGN, BSc, Dip N (Lond), RCNT, Dip N Ed (Lond), RNT*, former Director, Vocational Training, Bloomsbury and Islington College of Nursing and Midwifery, London.

Jenny Partridge, *BSc (Hons), RGN, Dip N (Lond)*, Teacher Facilitator, Department of Professional Development & Vocational Training, Frances Harrison College of Health Care, St Luke's Hospital, Guildford.

Jane Powell, *BSc (Hons) Nutrition, SRD*, Senior Dietitian for Older People, St Pancras Hospital, London.

Fay Reid, *BA, RN, Dip N (Lond), RNT, MSc, Certificate in Personnel Management*, Director of Patient Handling Courses, Bloomsbury and Islington College of Nursing and Midwifery, London.

Heather Rowe, *RN, BA, RNT, RCNT, Dip N (Lond)*, Nurse Teacher, Bloomsbury and Islington College of Nursing and Midwifery, London.

Dorothy Stables, *MSc, BA (Hons), RGN, RM, Dip N (Lond), MTD*, Senior Midwife Teacher/Course Director, St Bartholomew's College of Nursing and Midwifery, London.

Sue Whatton, *RNMH, Cert Ed*, Nurse Teacher, Hertfordshire College of Health Care Studies.

Lisa S. Whiting, *BA, RGN, RSCN, RNT, LTCL*, Nurse Teacher (Child Care), Barnet College of Nursing and Midwifery, Barnet.

Foreword
Jan Sutton, *SRN, SCM, ANA(H), Cert DMS*
Executive Director for Nursing & Patient Services
Wellhouse NHS Trust

Today's rapidly changing health care arena demands high levels of understanding and competence from all members of multi-disciplinary care teams. This book is a welcome addition to the, so far, relatively small number of texts available specifically relating to Health Care Assistants. The importance of understanding as a basis for confidence must not be underestimated in any caring role, particularly so in the emerging HCA role. The need to develop standards of care and work-based competency is paramount if quality patient/client care is to be achieved.

The authors and contributors to this book are experts in a wide range of health care fields. Using practical and authentic material they provide a clear guide to the expectations of those involved in giving support to professional practitioners, and also to those practitioners responsible for the management of Health Care Assistants. In the past there has been the temptation to describe care as a list of unlinked tasks. This book brings home the importance of understanding how care is planned and delivered in a patient-centred holistic manner. The challenges of change in health care can only really be achieved from this basis of understanding and competence.

The book is easily read and I particularly like the *Activity* notes involving readers in practical responses to the text. The book's three sections cover the range of care delivery in health institutions. The *Key words* at the beginning of each chapter clearly summarize its intent and are useful triggers for memory.

I am sure that the book will appeal to a wide audience within the health care field. Increasing importance is placed on the need for vocational training and qualifications, using work-based training, to prepare staff for assessment of competency and the award of National Vocational Qualifications. For the first time, staff delivering care but not involved in professional training, have the opportunity to validate their competency in a nationally recognized scheme. Those staff wishing to pursue these objectives will find *Knowledge to Care* of great value.

I know that those who work through this book will widen their horizons of understanding so that high quality patient care is maintained and developed.

I am grateful to the authors for broadening the knowledge base on the developing role of Health Care Assistants and, in so doing, providing this major source of practical advice and support to those engaged in patient care.

Editors' Acknowledgements

We are grateful to the contributors to this text for adding the materials concerning their particular areas of expertize and interest. We believe this will make the book of real value to our readers and assist them in providing high quality care.

Our thanks go to Jan Sutton for writing the Foreword, to Sharon Hartwell and Valerie Waller for their assistance with preparing the manuscript and to Ken Isaaks and Malcolm Johnson for permission to reproduce the photographs. Thanks are also due to the patients, clients and their families for permission to use the photographs.

We also wish to thank our colleagues, clients and ward staff for their cooperation and help, and the health care assistants who read through draft copies and enabled us to produce a text relevant to their needs.

We are grateful to the staff of Blackwell Science and especially to Lisa Field who asked us in the first place and then ensured that the book reached fruition.

Finally to the friends and families who provided support and did not complain at the price of time lost to them, we say
Thank You

Christine McMahon
Joan Harding

Introduction
Who the book is for and how to use it
Joan Harding

Care is about using *warmth, knowledge, understanding*, and *skill* to help another. Many have the capacity to care but lack the knowledge and skills to do so. *Knowledge to Care* aims to help provide the knowledge base from which those skills and awareness can be developed and enable carers to feel confident about what they do and how they do it.

Caring is usually a group activity, which needs organization and a leader. Care will usually be directed by professional practitioners of various disciplines, therefore care assistants assist in care and are responsible to these professionals.

Scope of care for health care assistants

The development of the health care assistant role as a support to professional practitioners of various disciplines is an important advancement in team approaches to care. It has significant implications for the quality of care delivered. It is also important that carers in this role recognize the value of vocational training to ensure that quality care is maintained.

Health care assistants work under the direction and supervision of registered practitioners, who remain accountable for the standards of care delivered and for determining the activity of their support staff, which must not be beyond their level of competence.

However, it cannot be said too often that support given by individuals who have acquired skill through knowledge and training can only enhance the quality of care given to individual clients. Therefore health care assistants should be encouraged and supported in obtaining vocational qualifications which recognize their skills, and these skills can be used for the benefit of their clients in a variety of settings.

We hope that this volume will be of value to:

Learners: Care assistants – as a source of information to act as a starting point for increasing knowledge and skill.
Teachers: As a resource in support of courses for health care assistants.
Patients and clients: Who will receive quality care from carers who have taken time to acquire knowledge and develop skills.

About This Book

On first opening a book a number of questions spring to mind. The information below is to help you decide whether this is the book you are looking for.

What is the book about?

It is about caring in health care settings.

Who is the book for?

It is written for health care assistants and those involved in caring in hospitals, residential homes, the community, or even looking after their own relatives or friends at home. *Knowledge to Care* is just that – it aims to provide information to help you understand the whys and wherefores of care for a range of patients or clients in a range of situations.

Is it about exams, tests or qualifications?

This is entirely up to you. If you are involved in preparing for assessment for NVQs (National Vocational Qualifications) the book will help you towards your goal. Alternatively, you may like to use it to enhance your understanding of the work you do each day. You may also find it helpful if you are involved in a caring course in a college or other institution.

How the book is presented

The book is divided into three major sections, each of which corresponds with a specific part of the framework of national care awards. Section 1 covers the Core Units for NVQs in Care; Section 2 deals with Endorsements for Direct/Acute Care and Section 3 is a selection of Endorsements for Care in specific situations, e.g. postnatal, the young child and care of the terminally ill client.

The book covers areas of care not dealt with in other available texts, and is primarily concerned with care given in health care institutions, though the principles may be applied in a variety of settings.

Each chapter has a group of *Key Words* at the beginning. These provide a brief indication of the content of the chapter and in particular, items or points to be remembered. Important words are italicized in the text to help you remember them, especially where they may not be familiar or are being used for the first time.

Activities

In each chapter you will find material headed *Activity* followed by a number. These are made to stand out from the rest of the text. Here you will be asked to stop and think, draw up a list, consider what you would do in certain circumstances, or discuss a topic with a colleague or colleagues. The whole aim of these *Activities* is to extend the range of material beyond the text of the chapter(s) and use your own thoughts, ideas or experiences. However, you may wish to read the chapter first and then return to the *Activities*. There is no right or wrong way, whatever you decide to do is right for you.

Did you know?

Also through the text you will find paragraphs with the heading '*Did you know?*' These are usually interesting snips of information, sometimes amusing, sometimes of historical interest. They are intended to help you remember certain items or facts. No doubt by the time you have finished the book and as a result of your own experiences, you will have thought of some *Did you knows?* of your own.

Finally, in order to help you locate the part of the book you most want at a particular time, there are a contents list, a comprehensive index and an appendix for matching up items in the text with units of the National Occupational Standards for NVQs in Care.

Section 1
Core Units for NVQs in Care

Chapter 1
Individuality and Sexuality of the Client
Christine McMahon and Francis Guilfoyle

Overview

This chapter introduces the client as an individual and helps us to understand the reasons for that individuality. When caring for a client there are many aspects of care that are integral in all we do for a specific client. This forms the basis of good practice and at all times it should reflect the following:

- The need for anti-discriminatory practice
- Recognizing the rights and choices of the client
- The importance of effective communication
- Maintaining the confidentiality of client information
- Recognizing the differences between all clients

You will find these statements of good practice reinforced throughout this book reflecting all aspects of care.

The chapter is in three sections; the first section helps us to understand how we formulate our ideas and attitudes, which are reflected in the way we behave and live out our lives. The middle section answers various questions concerning the sexuality of the client. These two sections will help to clarify why our clients may behave or act in certain ways and how conflict can occur in both the expectations of us towards clients and of clients' expectations of us as carers. The final section gives an explanation of how equal opportunities and access to care can be maintained.

Key words

Individual, values, beliefs, attitudes, culture, understanding, human concern, sexuality, lesbian, homosexual, equality, dignity, discrimination, rights, confidentiality, policy.

Making impressions and understanding others

First impressions

We are all separate *individuals* within society. The first impressions we formulate about our fellow human beings help us to understand this individuality. Many factors contribute to first impressions – outward appearance, manner or behaviour.

Activity 1.1 ■

 What do you notice when you meet someone for the first time? Write down your thoughts.

■ ■

You may have included:

- Sex
- Height
- Colour of eyes
- Facial expression

- Age
- Posture
- Skin texture
- Clothes that they are wearing

These are some of the things that I notice about someone I am meeting for the first time and this gives me an overall impression of them within seconds or minutes.

This impression will be influenced by my personal understanding of what I see, as this is *individual* to me alone. My perception of a person and situation will depend on my previous experiences which shape the way I interpret things that I see.

The context or situation will also influence my impression. For example should I see someone sitting in a dressing gown in a ward I would not consider this out of the ordinary (Fig. 1.1). But should I see the same person dressed in a dressing gown waiting for a bus on a cold and frosty morning, I would consider this to be out of the ordinary.

Fig. 1.1 Client within a care environment.

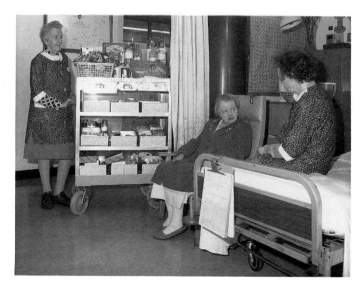

Fig. 1.2 Open position/ closed tense position.

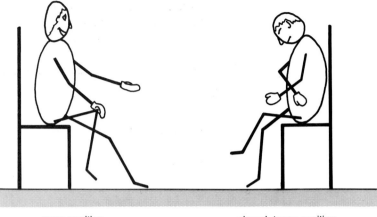

open position   closed, tense position

I may meet someone who is sitting in a chair smiling and looking up at me and with their shoulders relaxed and hands open. This would give me the impression that they are happy and relaxed and willing to communicate.

or

I may come up to someone who is sitting in a hunched up position, shoulders drawn up and hands clenched, and looking down. This would give me the impression this person is unhappy, perhaps in pain and not wishing to communicate with me. Figure 1.2 illustrates this particular example.

Factors affecting our impressions and attitudes

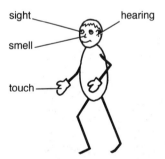

Fig. 1.3 First impressions are influenced by other senses as well as sight.

The visual first impression of a person is then reinforced or changed by using other senses as well as our sight (Fig. 1.3). For example speech and the way the person uses language, tone, inclination can give you lots of clues as to their level of understanding or mood. Touch can also indicate how someone is feeling, for example whether they feel confident as they shake your hand, and this could add to the first visual impression you had of their posture.

Many of the items that you listed display individuality and as a rule we have no control over them.

Activity 1.2 ■

Consider your list from Activity 1.1 and identify those items that you do not have any control over.

■ ■

These could include:

- Age
- Race
- And to some extent health

- Sex
- Culture

Throughout our lives there are influences that make us different. We all develop different *attitudes*, *values* and *beliefs*, and yet we also have many similarities that bind us together as a human race. Many influences help you to develop your values and beliefs and also socialize you. Your parents or guardians influenced you in your very early developmental years.

?

Did you know?

Japanese babies at the age of four months are physically passive and content just to watch people and things around them, whilst American babies are physically more active and vocal. This was found to reflect the distinct *cultural* differences; the Japanese *understand* babies to be separate and uncivilized beings who are brought into the family to be civilized. The Americans *understand* babies to be helpless and dependent, needing encouragement to develop and become independent and autonomous. (Caudill & Weinstein cited in Benner & Wrubel, 1989)

Activity 1.3 ■

As we develop and progress through life other people and situations influence us. Can you identify these?

■ ■

You may have thought of:

- Brothers and sisters
- Friends
- Environment and living conditions

- Grandparents
- Neighbours
- Clubs

and I am sure other factors

Our close family, parents/guardians, brothers, sisters and grandparents could all influence our behaviour (Fig. 1.4). And as our network develops to include peers and friends at school, neighbours, religious organizations, social clubs and, later, colleagues at work and people we meet socially, all these people help us to formulate our attitudes, beliefs and values.

The overall environment that we live in, poverty or affluence, any emotional trauma that we may have undergone and of course our cultures and beliefs will all influence our behaviour (Fig. 1.5). In addition the media, for example, newspapers, television, radio and theatre, may influence our *attitudes* and *values*. This results in the formation of our attitudes being influenced by others and at the same time we, in turn, are influencing their attitudes. This will affect our behaviour and initiate direct or indirect actions which could be positive or negative.

Fig. 1.4 Family group including great grandmother, grandparents and grand daughter.

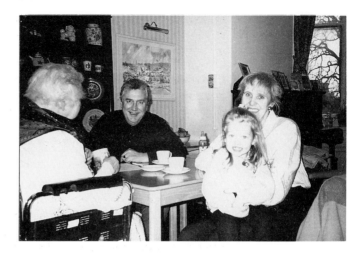

For example:

In some *cultures* it is not thought socially correct for a woman to expose certain areas of her body and much distress may be suffered should these areas need to be exposed for a medical examination. Client choice, rights and *culture* need to be both understood and respected in order to make a client feel valued and to obtain cooperation.

All individuals in society need to be aware of and respect others' role in life, culture and beliefs. We need to be able to adapt, cooperate and help others in order to live harmoniously. An individual who has come from a poor family and environment, being deprived of much by society, may feel that they have been treated unequally, with a resulting low self-esteem and a grudge against society. This may lead to anti-social behaviour. Treating such individuals with respect and consideration may alter their overall concept of society and have a favourable influence on their behaviour and their own self-esteem and worth.

Fig. 1.5 Factors which influence our behaviour.

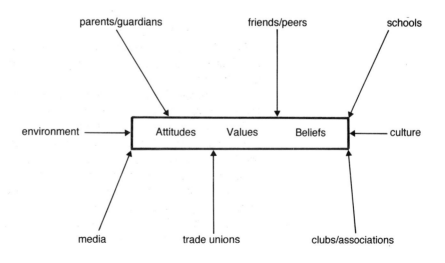

Categorizing other people

Background influences provided by culture, subculture and family all reflect in a person's behaviour. We are all results of our memberships of different groups, our relationships with different people and the variety of roles we play in life. Consequently we behave differently according to which group we are with or what role we are playing at that particular time.

Activity 1.4   ■

Consider the different roles in various groups you play in your life.

■ ■

These could be:

- Daughter/son
- Wife/husband
- Student
- Club member
- Chairperson of the local neighbours group

- Sister/brother
- Father/mother
- Employee
- Carer
- Choir member

We have expectations of others in specific roles and should these not conform to or not come up to our expectations, they can lead to conflicts and misunderstandings. We should be aware of this when we are caring for clients and not label them as 'different'. If a client has a disability we should not 'pigeon-hole' him or her as the 'one who is deaf' or the 'blind one'. We should always consider the whole person and not just concentrate on one particular characteristic, which in turn would put a person in a particular category and lead us to expect a certain type of behaviour.

For instance it is incorrect to think that fat people are jolly and rather lazy, and thin people are miserable and hard working (Fig. 1.6). This is a crude way of stereotyping and forming opinions of a person before we really get to know them and have some reason to back up our opinions.

How to treat a new client

On admission to a care environment a client may become more dependent as they enter the *patient role* and the carer plays the more dominant role, which in turn increases the client's dependency,.

When considering *individuality* one of the first things to take into account is what the client wishes to be called. It is important for you and other members of staff to clarify how clients wish to be addressed – whether it be a nickname, first name, or formal title such as Miss, Mrs or Mr.

Some clients may give you permission to use their first name. Others will prefer to use their marital status as an indication of how they like to be

Fig. 1.6 Thin and
miserable, fat and jolly.

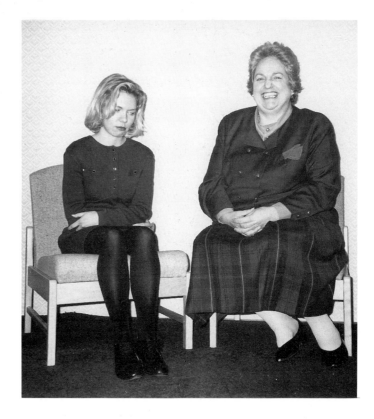

addressed. Do clarify this with the client. Many women who are divorced
may wish to use their maiden name.

It is often difficult for a person to find a suitable title for their partner if
they are not married, but living together. In this situation it is appropriate to
check with the client what they wish their partner to be called. Some clients
will have a partner of the same sex, and of course they must be given the
same rights and respects as any other spouse. This relationship may be a
homosexual one.

Client sexuality

Sexuality can mean different things to each individual and a variety of
approaches and attitudes to this topic is evident. This section of the chapter
is just one approach of many and gives the answers to some of the questions that you may wish to ask.

What do we mean by a homosexual relationship?

The term *homosexual* is used to describe a man or woman who prefers a sexual and emotional relationship with somebody of the same sex. A female homosexual relationship is known as a *lesbian* relationship.

How will I know if a client is a homosexual?

The only way you will know if a client is *gay* (a term often used to describe homosexual men) or lesbian is if they choose to share their feelings with you. When a client expresses feelings related to their sexual orientation, either heterosexual or homosexual, it is expected that you will respond in a manner which accepts the rights of this client and their chosen partner to good health care.

What if a client tells me something in confidence about their sexuality?

Do explain to the client that you feel it might be beneficial if they share this information with their doctor, but it must be the clients' choice to do this and not yours. You can offer to discuss this matter with the client, and their partner, and at the same time explain how sharing this information could benefit their health.

Why might a client want to discuss sexual matters with me?

It is often easier for someone to talk about intimate matters to a person who cares for them and whom they have learnt to trust; a person who can also give them time and privacy to listen to their fears and anxieties.

Very often diseases, surgery and sometimes drugs interfere with normal sexual feelings and functions. This can cause a great deal of stress to the client or their partner, putting a burden on the relationship. The fact that you are able actively to listen to somebody's problem will in itself be helpful, and will also enable you to seek help from others more experienced in dealing with sexuality problems. That is, with the client's permission of course.

I think I would find it difficult to talk about sex to a client

It is accepted that it is not always easy to talk about sexual issues. Clients will often use different terms to describe sexual activity and parts of their body. These could initially sound offensive but they may be the only words the person knows to describe the act of intercourse or that particular part of the body.

These words may have been learnt in the school playground, from parents or a biology book. Words such as *clap* instead of gonorrhoea (a sexually transmitted disease) or *my private parts* instead of penis or testicles are examples of how some people might use different words or expressions. The carer must always be sensitive about using sexual language or expressions that might offend others or cause confusion.

I think sexuality is very private and personal

This is why it is important to provide as much privacy as possible for clients and their partners. This privacy is respected when the client is attending to their toiletry needs, dressing or undressing. Their *privacy* and *dignity* must be preserved at all times.

Another need for privacy might be when the client wants to spend time alone with their partner; this might be for a matter of minutes or overnight, according to their sexual needs and general health at that particular time. This is very important when a couple are separated for some time because of the illness.

But not all clients are sexually active, are they?

Not all clients want to have, or enjoy sexual intercourse, but this is not the only way we express our sexuality. We often express our masculinity or femininity in other ways, such as by what we wear. Dressing in clothes that make us feel good is important to our well-being and self-esteem. Wearing make-up or perfume is another way women project their femininity. Men want to smell and look good according to their own personal ideals.

Many clients may require help in dressing and washing, especially in achieving good personal hygiene in order to feel comfortable. This is especially so if the client has problems with incontinence or is handicapped and has great difficulty in attending to their toiletry needs. Good personal hygiene promotes high self-esteem which is an important part of feeling good about our sexuality.

What about the client who wants to have sexual intercourse or enjoys masturbation?

This may be a consideration for the long-stay client in an institution or residential accommodation. This would be a situation that would require the client to have privacy in a safe and comfortable environment. There should be a *policy* as to how this need for privacy can be achieved in the best interest of the client, in order to prevent possible embarrassment to other clients or staff.

An open and honest dialogue with the client, partner and carers is essential in order to explore realistic ways that the client's sexual needs can be achieved, so that he or she can express them, taking into account the feelings and attitudes of those who have accepted the responsibility to care for the client.

Why do we want clients to express their sexuality?

To express our sexuality could be said to be a fundamental need of every individual, that when satisfied brings a feeling of well-being and contentment. It confirms our feelings of masculinity and femininity. If our sexual needs, like many other needs, are not fulfilled or are frustrated it can cause us to feel sad or even angry.

Even though the clients may be dependent on others, and on us for their care, we hope to be able to help them express their sexuality according to their own personal *beliefs* and *ethics*.

Equal opportunities and access to care

In this final section the principles of *equality* will be discussed. Many organizations' standards of care and *policies* reflect the *Patients' Charter* (Department of Health, 1992), especially within the health care setting. In order to treat all clients equally we must always be aware of the risk of *discriminating* between one client and another. Discrimination can appear in different ways and some examples will be discussed in the following sections.

Direct discrimination

This happens when a person or a group of people are treated less favourably than others in the same situation. For example, clients who are confined to a wheelchair and, due to the lack of ramps in place of steps, are restricted from entering certain areas, such as the hospital shop or chapel. Therefore access must be equal for everyone.

Activity 1.5 ■

Consider your work area – can clients and their visitors get everywhere? Are there lifts, ramps and wide doorways to allow free access to public areas?

■ ■

Indirect discrimination

This occurs when a specific requirement or condition is unfair or unjust. For example, in order to have clean clothes all clients must have someone who is able to take any soiled clothing home to wash and maintain a constant supply of clean clothes. Have you facilities for washing and ironing personal clothing in your organization?

Institutional discrimination

This occurs when particular policies, practices or procedures have a discriminatory effect on someone. For example, an organization may not have any facilities for providing food for vegetarians. This would discriminate against those clients who do not eat meat and their choice of food would be restricted.

Activity 1.6 ■

Have you ever cared for a client who was a vegetarian? If so what diet was available for them?

■ ■

Main factors of discrimination

- Disability, whether physical or mental
- Sex, sexual orientation
- Social status
- Race, colour, national ethnic origin
- Religion, creed

There are certain Acts of Parliament that have been passed and it is from these that health authorities, hospital trusts and organizations formulate their policies and guidelines for good practice. You should be familiar with your own organization's policies, concerning for example equal opportunities, employment and health and safety policies. These are based on the Sex Discrimination Act, Race Relations Act, Disabled Persons Act and the Health and Safety at Work Act.

You should be familiar with the Acts and policies that apply to your own work area, for example the Mental Health Act for those who work in the mental health field. It is your responsibility to keep up to date with any new policies or procedures that could affect the way in which you care for your own client group.

Activity 1.7 ■

List the policies that relate to your specific work area; are they readily accessible for reference?

■ ■

An equal opportunities policy should reflect a positive outlook for clients and value them in order for them to maintain their self-esteem and individuality. All cultural groups should be catered for in order to ensure equal access to treatment and care.

Activity 1.8 ■

Make a list of what could appear in an equal opportunities policy for your organization.

■ ■

Your list might include:

- Information
- Privacy and dignity
- Food that reflects individual beliefs and culture
- Special facilities for relatives and friends
- Confidentiality
- Health promotion
- Care for the dying that considers religion and culture
- Choice of carers

Information

This is one of the most important aspects of care as *fear of the unknown* impedes recovery, makes it more difficult for a client to cope with pain and can generally increase the dependence of the client on others for care. In addition, lack of information may result in the client not being fully aware of their *rights of care*, *aids for living* or *supplementary benefits*.

Information can be linked with power; those with information can be in a more powerful position than those with limited access to information. Information should be shared, with equal access for all clients and their relatives and friends. All information should be available in different languages, sign language, braille and symbols, in order to meet the needs of client groups. A patient advocacy and interpreting service should be available and the carer should know how and when to contact them.

Confidentiality

All clients, their relatives and friends should be guaranteed *confidentiality* of information that they wish to disclose to all grades of carers. This is closely linked to privacy and *dignity*. It is an essential aspect of care and a basic need of clients to make them feel safe in their environment, and it does in turn show that we both respect and value them as *individuals*. Examples of confidential information were discussed in the previous section, on client sexuality.

All records pertaining to the client are confidential and must be kept in a safe place and access only allowed to those who are authorized to read them (Fig. 1.7). All clients are now allowed access to medical records that have been written since November 1991. Each organization has a procedure to follow should clients wish to read their own notes.

Complaints procedure

All our clients and their relatives should be aware of the organization's complaints procedure should they wish to lodge a complaint. If complaints are attended to swiftly and thoroughly then clients will feel that the organization cares for them as individuals and that standards of care are maintained.

Fig. 1.7 Sharing information.

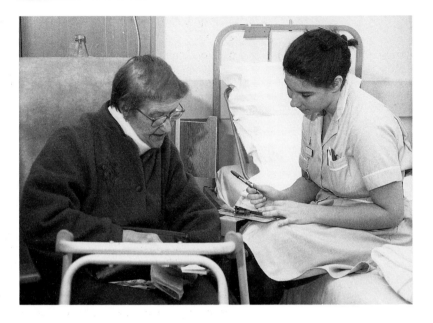

Activity 1.9 ■

 Are you aware of your own organization's procedure? If not obtain a copy and read it through.

■ ■

Health promotion and education

This should apply to and be available for not only people directly in our care but also for the local community. To ensure equal access to all it should be available in different languages and braille. It should identify specific needs and motivate self-care and independence of the individual.

Bereavement and care of the terminally ill

Each client should have their individual wishes met concerning their cultural and religious beliefs in death and dying. You should be aware of the most common religious and cultural needs of your client group and where you can obtain more detailed information and help from religious leaders.

Catering

Food should be acceptable to all client groups and in accordance with their individual preferences. As food and nutrition are such important aspects of life, both physically and socially every effort should be made to ensure clients are given food of their choice, provided it is not contraindicated.

Activity 1.10 ■

List the clients with different religious beliefs that you have cared for. How were their specific needs met concerning diet, death.

■ ■

Privacy and dignity

Every client should be guaranteed privacy for personal care. Curtains or screens should be adequate and always used. Separate facilities in surroundings that meet individual needs should be available for males and females. For example, in out-patients or X-ray departments gowns should be available that completely cover the client. Help in fastening the gowns should be readily available if necessary.

Choice of carers

There may be times when a client wishes to choose a carer of a particular sex. For instance a woman who has been raped may prefer to be cared for by a female. A nun or a Muslim woman may also wish to be cared for by a female. Otherwise clients should not refuse care from a carer on grounds of their sex, race or colour, but should consider the skill and expertize of the carer instead.

It is important to explain to the client who will be carrying out investigations. For some females it may be difficult to accept that they will receive care from a male, especially in the case of vaginal examinations, and the opportunity for explanation must be made available. This may be at times in the form of counselling.

Facilities for relatives and friends

Private quiet areas should be available for relatives or friends, especially of the very ill clients. There should be somewhere visitors can rest and stay overnight should they so wish. This should also be available for parents with young children who are in hospital. Crèche, feeding and nappy changing facilities should also be available for mothers of babies and young children.

Summary

In this chapter we have concentrated on why each of us and our clients are *individuals* and how this individuality can be both respected and maintained. Questions have been answered concerning aspects of *sexuality*. References have been made to various *legislation* and organizational *policies* that facilitate care and make us all aware of the individual needs of our clients, irrespective of their sex, race, creed, sexual orientation or physical disability. For the policies to be effective, all the carers and other staff within the organization must give their personal commitment.

References

Benner, P. & Wrubel, J. (1989) *The Primacy of Caring*, p. 46. Addison-Wesley Publishing Company, California.
Department of Health (1992) *Patients' Charter*. HMSO, London.

Further reading

Your own local organizational policies concerning:

- Anti-discrimination and anti-racist practices;
- Health and safety at work;
- Equal opportunities;

- Relevant Acts and organizational policies;
- Ward or departmental philosophy of care.

Allen, C. (1992) Sexuality matters. *Nursing Times*, 12 August, **88**(33), 22.
Canis, P. (1992) Attending the spirit. *Nursing Times*, 5 August, **88**(32), 50.
Crowley, J. (1991) Races apart. *Nursing Times*, 10 March, **87**(10), 44–6.
Green, S. (1991) A two faced society. *Nursing Times*, 14 August, **87**(33), 26–9.
Hendrick, J. (1991) Acting for children. *Nursing Times*, 24 April, **87**(17), 64–6.
Holmes, P. (1991) Advocacy, the patient's friend. *Nursing Times*, 8 May, **87**(19), 16–17.
Messenger, K. (1992) *Clients as Individuals*. Churchill Livingstone, Edinburgh.
Moore, K. (1991) Confronting taboo. *Nursing Times*, 16 October, **87**(42), 46–7.
Neilan, S. (1991) Careless words. *Nursing Times*, 20 November, **87**(47), 52–3.
Parke, F. (1991) Sexuality in later life. *Nursing Times*, 11 December, **87**(50), 40–42.
Savage, J. (1987) *Nurses, Gender and Sexuality*. Heinemann, London.
Sillars, S. (1992) *Caring for People*, pp. 51–3. Macmillan, Basingstoke.

Chapter 2
Communications
Jenny Partridge

Overview

The art of communication is of great importance in a care setting and in this chapter the different methods of communication are discussed, concentrating on verbal and non-verbal methods. The barriers to communication are described, including perception and the environment.

Key words

Verbal, non-verbal, sensory deficit, interpersonal skills, personal presentation, aids to communication, team working, perception, environment.

What is communication?

We all talk about communication, but what do we actually mean? To start with, try and define what you mean by communication.

Activity 2.1 ■■■■■■■■■■■■■■■■■■■■■■■■■■■

 Identify six words which would answer the question: 'What does communication mean to you?

■■■■■■■■■■■■■■■■■■■■■■■■■■■■■■

You may have used words such as:

- Information
- Speaking
- One person to another
- Writing

Let's look at the *Oxford English Dictionary*: 'The imparting or exchange of information'. This is a broad definition of communication, which is constantly necessary for us to manage our everyday lives. Information can be misunderstood and misinterpreted very easily and the consequences of this can be devastating, especially in the health care environment.

When do we start communicating?

Some scientists would say that a baby in the womb is capable of receiving communications and that behaviour patterns after birth reflect messages sent by their mothers.

So how do we communicate?

Often communication is broken down into two broad categories: *verbal* and *non-verbal*.

Activity 2.2 ■

Find some examples of verbal communication.

■ ■

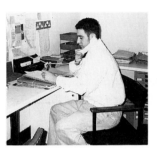

Fig. 2.1 Communicating on the telephone.

For *verbal* communication you might have written speech and talking and then got stuck. You may have extended the list to include television and radio. If you think of verbal meaning words then your list may suddenly have grown to include newspapers, magazines, letters, telephones, faxes, electronic mail, etc.

The way that you speak can be examined in terms of tone, pitch and speed, for example, which are all parts of speech and are called para-linguistics. Also 'hm hm' and 'uh uh' act as reinforcement for communications. All the time words are being delivered as a means of communicating. This may be a two- way communication, such as talking to someone face to face or on the telephone (Fig. 2.1), or one-way, such as looking at television or reading the newspaper.

Activity 2.3 ■

List some examples of non-verbal communication.

■ ■

Examples of *non-verbal* communication that you may have identified could be:

- Eye contact
- The distance you stand away from the person with whom you are communicating and whether you are sitting or standing and level with each other
- Facial expressions
- Body language, for example the way you stand, place your hands or arms, gestures
- Touch

In fact these are as important if not more important than the verbal examples.

Body language

This is a large subject and can be broken down into a number of smaller areas. The overall picture presented to someone else is very important. The first and last impressions that people have of you are the ones that they remember – the *primary* and *recency* effects, as psychologists like to call them. Consequently *personal presentation* is an important part of communication.

Verbal and non-verbal communications should reflect or reinforce each other. Imagine how you would feel as a client if a carer asked you how you were feeling and they were standing with their arms crossed and did not meet your eye?

Or

You asked a client how they were feeling and they said fine, but when you observed them they were curled up in bed with downcast eyes. In both these examples two different messages are being given.

What sort of impression do you wish to give to your client? The position of our bodies is most important and will communicate a great deal to our companion(s). If someone is leaning forward it tends to signify interest and encouragement, whilst leaning backwards could be interpreted as boredom or disinterest, or on the other hand extreme relaxation. Equally, crossed arms may indicate a lack of interest and not wishing to get involved, even though it may be a cold day and you are trying to keep warm! These closed signals can also indicate a wish to terminate the conversation as quickly as possible and go on to something else.

Eye contact

Lovers are described as 'gazing into each other's eyes', but too much eye contact can be disconcerting and lead to discomfort on the part of the recipient. The eyes are said to be the 'mirror of the soul' and messages are sent unconsciously to the other person. When we are listening to someone we tend to maintain eye contact (Fig. 2.2), but when we are speaking we tend to have intermittent eye contact and signals can be sent to indicate 'I'm ready to speak or listen'.

Activity 2.4 ■

Without telling a colleague what you are going to do, carry on a conversation with them for two minutes keeping close eye contact. Then continue the conversation with them for another two minutes deliberately avoiding any eye contact. How do you both feel at the end?

■ ■

Probably your colleague will ask what on earth you were doing, but will also say that they felt quite threatened in the first exercise and it was difficult

Fig. 2.2 Maintaining eye contact.

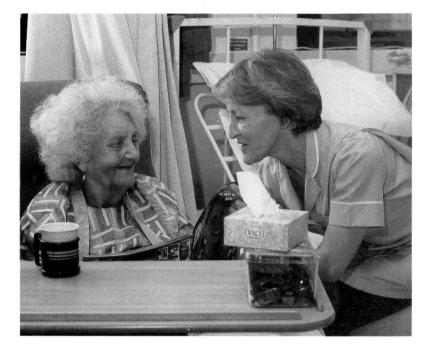

to keep the conversation going. In the second the comments may well be that you appeared disinterested and weren't really concerned with what was being said.

Eye contact can reinforce the messages that we are sending. However it may have particular significance in different cultures. In some cultures it is considered discourteous to look someone in the eye if they are older or wiser than yourself.

Position and space

Linked to eye contact is the comparative position we place ourselves in to communicate.

Activity 2.5 ■■■■■■■■■■■■■■■■■■■■■■■■■■■■

Try placing yourself in different positions relative to your colleague and carry on a conversation. These positions may be side by side, one standing and one sitting, back to back, very close together and wide apart, for example. You will probably think of more. Which were the easiest?

■■■■■■■■■■■■■■■■■■■■■■■■■■■■■■■■■■

You will probably have found sitting nearly opposite to each other the easiest and the distance may well reflect the length of time you have known each other. The better we know a person the nearer we let them come to us. We have an 'intimate area' which is approximately 18 inches around

facing each other

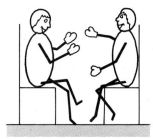

confrontational

side by side

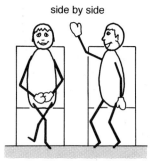

sharing

at an angle of 45°

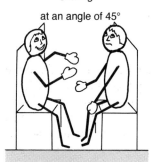

this position gives the
person the opportunity to
maintain or break eye
contact as they wish

Fig. 2.3 Communication.

us, a 'personal area' from there to about four feet, then a 'social area' up to 12 feet and finally a public area from there onwards (Marsh, 1988).

On the whole we do not allow anyone to violate our personal space, or we have strict conditions if this happens. As carers we have to gain permission to enter that intimate zone as so much of our care is very personal and does in fact violate that space.

Activity 2.6 ■

When you are in a queue, for example waiting for a bus or a checkout in a supermarket, see what happens if you edge forward nearer the next person. Be careful about the supermarket trolleys!

■ ■

The chances are that the person you tried to get nearer to tried to get away and keep the ratio of space the same. You may also have been the recipient of some fairly foul glances as well – another method of *non-verbal* communication and protection of space.

Relative position

This is also important in the physical levels of people; if one person is much higher than the other it can be seen as a commanding position and the lower person feels at a disadvantage. It can also hinder or facilitate eye contact and effective communication.

We can also send messages to the client by changing our relative position. For example if we sit down to talk to a client it is telling them we have time and will concentrate on them for that specific time.

Emphasis on words

The emphasis we put on words can also hinder or improve communication. It can also alter the meaning of what was meant to be said.

Activity 2.7 ■

Think of a simple sentence such as 'This is my pen'. Emphasize each word in turn and see how different meanings can be constructed.

■ ■

You could alter the tone in which you speak the words and see what reactions you get from others.

Gestures

These are often used to emphasize points. Some people use gestures more than others, and continue to gesture to emphasize points when they are on

Fig. 2.4 Interaction zones (adapted from Hall in Hargie & Saunders, 1987).

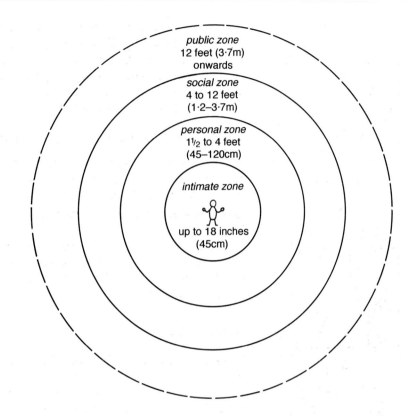

public zone
12 feet (3·7m)
onwards

social zone
4 to 12 feet
(1·2–3·7m)

personal zone
1½ to 4 feet
(45–120cm)

intimate zone

up to 18 inches
(45cm)

the telephone, even though their listener cannot see them. On the other hand gestures can also signal what the body really feels rather than what is being said (Argyle & Trower, 1979). If you watch someone who is being interviewed they may appear calm and say they are not worried, but in fact they are fiddling with something or crossing and uncrossing their legs all the time. So messages may be contrary in their presentation and the true reaction has to be found for effective communication to take place.

Smiling and nodding one's head are encouragements to others to continue to talk. Smiling alters the tone of the voice and it is suggested that you should smile whilst answering the telephone as it sounds better the other end. It will give confidence to someone to continue and put over their point of view. It also reinforces the fact that you are interested and listening to the client. A useful way you can remember this is:

SOLER: Smile
          Open manner
          Lean forward
          Eye contact
          Relax

(adapted from Egan, 1985).

Fig. 2.5 Gestures reinforcing communication.

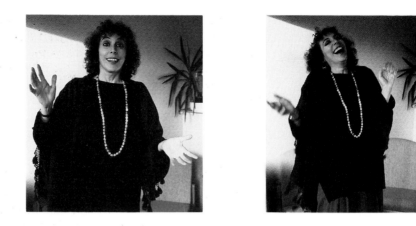

Touch

There are times when it may be said that gestures speak louder than words. The way that we handle or touch clients can be a positive way of communication and our attitude can be portrayed in the way that we may lift a client's leg when washing or turning them. I am sure when you have felt upset someone may have just touched your arm or squeezed your hand and no words are necessary to tell you that the other person cares.

Barriers to communication

Having reviewed different methods of communication we can see where problems may arise in messages and intentions being understood and acted upon appropriately. The saying goes that, 'You can take a horse to water but you cannot make it drink'.

The same is true for communication; you can tell someone something but they may not act upon it for a variety of reasons. It may be a simple reason of not hearing and a straight repetition will ensure the intended response. Or the reasons may be more complex. The hearer may not wish to act on that communication, so even if they hear the words they won't do anything about it deliberately.

There may be a physical reason for the communication gap. *Sensory deprivation* such as deafness, blindness, learning difficulties or illness may lead to barriers being put in the way. Or in the multicultural society in which we now live, there may be a language barrier.

Blindness

Activity 2.8 ■

 Working with a partner, take turns in putting a blindfold on and being led round the classroom by the 'sighted' partner.

■ ■

You probably felt very disorientated despite the fact you thought you knew where you were, and you asked a great many questions of your partner about where you were and where pieces of furniture were. In communication we use a number of senses to understand messages and once we lose one of those senses we need additional information and reassurance to maintain the same level of understanding.

Deafness

Activity 2.9 ■

Again, working with a partner, ensure they cannot hear by using a personal stereo or equivalent and then ask them to undertake a simple task such as moving a book from one table to another, without demonstrating. How successful is the 'deaf' person?

■ ■

Hearing loss is often described as the unseen handicap as people look normal but yet appear to have difficulty in comprehending information. It therefore becomes an enormous communication barrier unless people adapt their behaviour to cope with this.

If people suffer hearing loss, in addition to having an aid, learning sign language or lip reading if their loss is severe, they develop *coping strategies* for enhancing their level of understanding. If the speaker's face is clearly lit, and turned upwards, this helps the deaf individual to lip read and follow facial expressions. The speaker should also speak clearly and reasonably slowly so that the deaf person has a better chance of hearing. Deaf people often tip their heads in the direction of the speaker in order to try and hear more clearly and block out *extraneous noise*.

Speech disorders

The inability to speak is another barrier to communication. This could, for example, be due to a stroke resulting in dysphasia (difficulty in speaking). There are many clients who have a speech disorder and who may exhibit great frustration in attempting to communicate. The speech therapist plays an important role in assessing and treating these clients.

Learning difficulties and language barriers

Barriers are evident if people have learning difficulties. As we develop, our brain's ability to understand and comprehend expands. It is beyond a child's capability to understand what time is until they have learned to tell the time, so communication has to be altered for them to understand. Even so as adults we are guilty of saying to clients that we will be there 'in a minute' whilst there is not the slightest chance that we can be there in under a quarter of an hour.

Communication then has to reflect the common ground and abilities between the parties involved and sometimes this requires the asking of questions to identify the common ground. Use of language varies from limited to extended. At times limited language may be necessary – for example if someone is in danger we may just call out 'Stop', but if there is no danger and we want someone's attention to talk to them we may say, 'Hang on a minute will you, I'd like to have a word'.

Questioning

Activity 2.10 ■

Write down all the types of or ways of asking questions you can think of.

■ ■

The list is probably quite extensive and may include the following:

- Open
- Factual
- Clarifying
- Leading

- Closed
- Rhetorical
- Multiple

There is a place for all these types of questions in communication, but they must be used in the appropriate way to be effective and careful thought must be given before using the last two, as they either confuse or control communications.

By getting answers to questions, it is possible to judge whether there are barriers there that need to be overcome.

Open questions

These encourage a full answer and the respondent has a chance to put forward their comments, feelings and opinions.

Closed questions

These, on the other hand, are used when a brief response is required and may link with factual questions where the questioner is trying to elicit responses for factual purposes. They are usually answered by a 'yes' or 'no'.

Rhetorical questions

These are used when it could be thought that the client wants to talk more, and by repeating the statement in a questioning manner the respondent may speak further.

Clarifying questions

These may use the same structure to ensure that the questioner and respondent are talking about the same thing and putting similar meanings to the subject.

Multiple questions

These are very tempting to ask, especially if there is a time constraint involved. However it is very difficult for the respondent to reply as there is a large degree of uncertainty as to which answer belongs to which question!

Leading questions

These tend to invite a specific answer and the respondent may feel under pressure to give the expected answer rather than the one which they will really want to give. These questions can be used when enquiring about someone's well-being. For instance we may say 'Feeling all right are you?' and the expected answer is 'Yes, thank you'.

Language

The variety of languages you can encounter in our society today means that we require either an excellent interpreting service or some other means of making sure we are communicating effectively. *Language cards* are one solution, and language cards with pictures are even better, given the wide variety of dialects involved.

Even in English, word meanings alter in different parts of the country and there are different words to describe even the most simple of actions. It is a challenge to find the appropriate word, but much distress can be avoided if this is realized early.

Not only is language different, but gestures which are quite usual and normal in one country can be perceived as being rude and insulting in another. For example in the Middle East it is considered polite to burp at the end of the meal to signify appreciation of the food you have eaten, and not to is an insult to the host.

Colloquial expressions also cause consternation to people who are learning English as their second language. How many times have you asked someone to 'hang on' at the other end of the telephone? Hang on to what?

Every type of work has its own jargon; perhaps in the caring services we have even more, or our time is at a premium so we use jargon as a short cut. Again it does mean that everyone should have an understanding of what the jargon actually means, and preferably for reasons of safety it should be used as little as possible.

Activity 2.11   ■

Make a list of all the jargon terms you can find in your place of work.

■ ■

No examples are going to be given here, but do you truly know the meaning of all the words in *your* list? If not, ask at least one other person for definitions and don't use the word(s) in the meantime.

As an individual every client will have differing communication needs. As a carer you will need to use your skills to find the most appropriate and effective methods of communicating with your clients. Equally, you have a responsibility to communicate within your team. *Team work* is made up of a great many lines of communication and if these are broken or inadequately maintained the wrong messages may get through.

Activity 2.12   ■

Make a list of all the team members with whom you communicate during a span of duty.

■ ■

Fig. 2.6 Some members of the caring team.

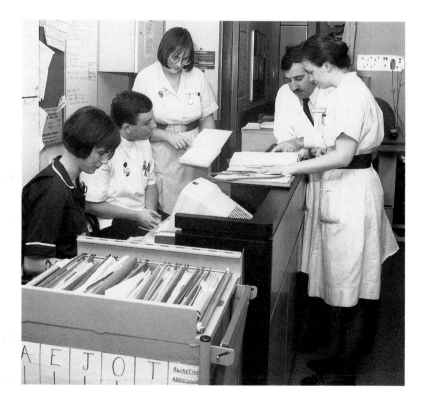

You may only have a small list if you work mainly on your own or in a small team. However if you work in a large busy hospital you may have a very long list. Figure 2.6 shows some team members. Whatever the size, all communication is important.

Other factors affecting communication

Physical/psychological

How we are feeling at any one time will affect communication. If you feel happy then you feel like chatting freely; however if you are in pain or discomfort then you may not feel like talking to anyone at all.

Perception

This is our personal understanding or interpretation and it is dependent on previous experiences. Perception is two-way and while we perceive the person with whom we are communicating, they are perceiving us. There are times when we need to check our perception. For instance, if we see someone curled up in bed looking unhappy, we may wish to check by asking 'How are you feeling?', or by saying 'I get the impression that you're feeling fed up and may be in some sort of discomfort'. Hopefully this will let the client know that you are receiving their message and are concerned about them.

Environment

The overall environment can either inhibit or facilitate communication.

Activity 2.13 ■

List factors in the environment that could inhibit communication.
■ ■

Such factors could include:

- Noise
- Table in between two people
- Seating arrangements

Activity 2.14 ■

List factors in the environment that could facilitate communication.
■ ■

Fig. 2.7 Sharing information – sitting on chairs of equal height.

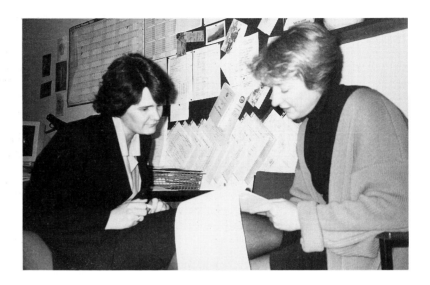

The factors could include:

- Comfortable chairs set at an angle and at the same height (Fig. 2.7)
- Soft light
- Quietness

Summary

This chapter has looked at communication. Consider the *Activities* you have completed. You are now ready to look for opportunities to enhance your communication skills in all aspects of caring.

References

Argyle, M. & Trower, P. (1979) *Person to Person; Ways of Communicating.* Harper & Row, London.

Egan, G. (1985) *The Skilled Helper, a Systematic Approach to Effective Helping.* Brooks/Cole Publishing Company, California.

Marsh, P. (1988) *Eye to Eye; How People Interact.* Salem House Publishers, Massachusetts.

Further reading

Anderson, M. (1992) *I'm the Same as You.* Available from Care group manager for people with learning difficulties, Hull Community Health, Victoria House, Park Street, Hull HU2 8TD.

Hargie, O., Saunders, C. & Dickson, D. (1987) *Social Skills in Interpersonal Communication.* Croom Helm, London.

Hodges, D. (1992) Can you hear me? *Nursing Times*, 1 July, **88**(27), 41.

Lloyd, A. (1991) Stop, look and listen. *Nursing Times*, 20 March, **87**(12), 30.

Marrion, M. (1992) Taking on Alfie. *Nursing Times*, **88**(33), 36–7.

Neilan, S. (1991) Careless words. *Nursing Times*, 20 November, **87**(47), 52–3.

Phillips, J. (1992) Breaking down barriers. *Nursing Times*, 26 August, **88**(35), 30–31.

Scammell, B. (1990) *Communication Skills.* Macmillan, London.

Tolson, D. & Swan, I. (1991) Facing up to deafness. *Nursing Times*, 5 June, **87**(23), 26.

Waterman, H. & Webb, C. (1992) Visually impaired patients' perceptions of their needs in hospital. *Nursing Practice*, **5**(3), 6–9.

Wilkinson, S. (1992) Confusions and challenges. *Nursing Times*, 26 August, **88**(35), 24–8.

Williams, N. (1991) Meaningful dialogue. *Nursing Times*, 23 January, **88**(4), 52–3.

Chapter 3
Managing Difficult Behaviour
Caroline Coleman and Sue Whatton

Overview

This chapter will look at difficult behaviour and its management. First a definition is offered about how and why difficult behaviour happens, followed by an explanation of how to deal with situations when they occur, and their aftermath. Emphasis is laid on recording and reporting such events. Finally a case study is included to help in the application of principles of managing difficult behaviour.

Key words

Behaviour, feelings, reaction, cause, trigger, records, policies, procedure, observation, de-brief, awareness, limitations.

What is difficult behaviour?

The term 'difficult behaviour' is extremely hard to define. As we are all individuals our perception of what is difficult behaviour will vary enormously from person to person. Our responses and coping strategies will differ as much as our perceptions. For this reason it is fair to say that difficult behaviour may be any *behaviour* that makes you feel uncomfortable, worried or frightened. It may also be a behaviour which is new to you, which you have not witnessed before and therefore do not know how to cope or deal with. What may appear trivial to one person may seem difficult to another, depending on our knowledge, skills and past experience. It is important to recognize this so that we can be open and supportive within our working team.

Activity 3.1 ■

 Describe one example of a recent incident in which you experienced behaviour which you felt was difficult.

■ ■

Here are some examples of difficult behaviour:

- When out shopping, the shop assistant ignored me
- On my way to work, I bumped into a man walking along the road and he swore at me
- Yesterday morning whilst serving breakfast, a new patient threw her cereal at me

Within the working environment, difficult behaviour from a client is obstructive and upsetting for the carer. At the least it incurs *feelings* of frustration and fear, at the worst physical injury. Difficult behaviour is often unexpected and, without preparation, response to that behaviour may be inappropriate and emotional.

Carers can find themselves in a position of risk, often because, however unprepared, they feel they have to act. With adequate preparation and training, carers should become competent in assessing a situation and acting objectively and appropriately in dealing with a problem as it occurs. No-one can guarantee a 100% success rate, but the risk factor can certainly be reduced significantly.

Activity 3.2   ■

How did you react to the difficult behaviour you described in Activity 3.1. How did you feel about the incident?

■ ■

Examples of answers may be:

- *I reacted by*   getting cross and tutting;
  walking away quickly;
  standing still with my mouth open.
- *I felt*   angry and frustrated;
  frightened;
  surprised and shocked.

Why does difficult behaviour happen?

There are many factors which may *trigger* difficult behaviour and usually in the course of our work we will not witness the cause of the *behaviour*, but we may act as the trigger. The *cause* is the underlying reason why a person is likely to present difficult behaviour. The trigger is the factor that initiates the actual behaviour. It is important, therefore, that we are aware of our own patterns of behaviours and how others may react to them. The causes/triggers are often confused but both can fall in to three main categories which may overlap each other. These categories are physical, psychological and environmental, and examples are given under each heading (Table 3.1).

Table 3.1 Causes/triggers of difficult behaviour.

Physical	Psychological	Environmental
Pain	Emotional upsets	Room temperature
Dietary factors	Stress	Unjustified restrictions
Alcohol/drugs	Tension	Noise
Hunger/thirst	Confusion	Unknown surroundings
Hormonal	Frustration	Unfamiliar persons
Clinical conditions	Powerless	Others' behaviour
Shock	History of abuse	Routine changes

Activity 3.3 ■

Refer back to your initial answers in Activities 3.1 and 3.2. To test your understanding, list possible triggers of the difficult behaviours you described.

■ ■

Examples of answers may be:

- Emotional upset
- Noise
- My behaviour/approach

Activity 3.4 ■

Apply these principles to clients you may have cared for in a hospital or residential situation and identify possible constraints which might lead to difficult behaviour.

■ ■

Possible constraints may include:

- Lack of privacy
- Crowding
- Lack of freedom and choice
- Boredom
- Lack of understanding of what is happening to them
- Insufficient stimulation or individual attention

Activity 3.5 ■

Anger may be a very real part of difficult behaviour. Make a list of signs which may indicate that a client's level of anger is increasing.

■ ■

Your list might include:

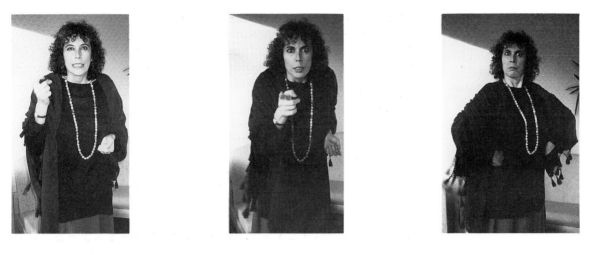

Fig. 3.1 Visual indications of a person's mood, reflecting anger and indignation.

- Tension in body posture
- Grim facial expression
- Increased volume and rate of speech

- Clenched fists
- Grinding of teeth
- Abusive language
- Violent behaviour

Figure 3.1 illustrates visual indications of anger and indignation.

How do we deal with difficult behaviour?

Meeting difficult behaviour with difficult behaviour:

- Prolongs the episode
- Risks your job

- Increases the risk of injury

The best method of dealing with difficult behaviour is to make sure that you are well prepared before the incident occurs. Take some time to think about how prepared you would be in dealing with a difficult situation. Listed below are some guidelines to help you prepare:

- Whenever possible get to know your client. Try to make time to read new client's admission or care plan documents.
- Find out if *training and updating* is available and ask to participate.

- Discuss with your colleagues how they would feel about being faced with difficult behaviour. Talk about how they would respond. Share experiences.
- Ask senior staff for guidance and find out which *policies* and *procedures* are appropriate.

- Find out if there are any code signals which make other staff aware that you are in difficulty.

- Be aware of your approach and the effect it may have on others.

Example of dealing with difficult behaviour

The incident described below illustrates some features of difficult behaviour and how they might be dealt with.

> Sally is a care assistant working in out-patients. One morning, Bill arrives at the department to have his hearing aid checked. As he comes through the door he is screaming. Sally approaches him and notices his breath smells of alcohol. Sally approaches him with a calm manner, and he lurches towards her. She takes one step back and gently asks if she can help. Bill continues to swear and shouts that he has a loud noise in his head. Sally asks if Bill would like to sit down whilst she gets someone to help him, but he ignores her. Sally's voice remains calm and she continues by telling Bill that she will phone the doctor to come and see him about the pain in his head. Bill sits down and begins to calm down. Sally goes to the phone and summons help by using a pre-arranged code word during her phone conversation.
>   If Sally had not remained calm the outburst could have become prolonged, dangerous and time-consuming.

Observation of potentially difficult clients

If you are caring for a client who you know has difficult behaviour and you are not sure what may be causing this, in preparation for future incidents it is likely that you and other colleagues may be asked to *observe* that client.

There are several ways to observe people. The most obvious way is just to keep an extra close eye on them, but the results may be influenced by the individual carer's own perceptions. The most reliable way is to record behaviour observed using a recognized and agreed observation chart. Never document observed behaviour without the agreement of senior staff.

The *observation chart* most commonly used and recognized is the ABC chart (Fig. 3.2), which is based on:

A   Antecedent – what happened before the incident;
B   Behaviour – what behaviour was observed;
C   Consequence – what happened immediately after the incident.

From observations recorded on a form as described for a prescribed period of time you will probably see a pattern emerge.

Example:
Every time the client is offered breakfast he becomes difficult. This cue is for you to discover why breakfast is a problem?

Fig. 3.2 ABC observation chart (adapted from the *STEP Manual*).

Day/time	Antecedent	Behaviour observed	Consequences	Signature

Activity 3.6 ■

 Using Table 3.1, list some possible reasons for the difficult behaviour to occur at breakfast time.

■ ■

You may have answers like this:
The client was always offered bacon and eggs and the client is Jewish and does not eat meat from the pig.

or

The carer who brought the breakfast always ignored the client and refused to acknowledge the client's existence.

or

The doctor had told the client that they must have their tablets immediately after eating. The drug round always came some time after breakfast had been served and cleared away. The client waited for the drugs to be given before eating and therefore breakfast was cold.

What to do when an incident occurs

However well prepared you may be, unpredictable or difficult behaviour may still occur. Faced with difficult situations you should not just let things carry on until they become unmanageable. There are two main ways to respond appropriately:

(1) Deal with the incident;
(2) Go away and get help.

The option you choose will depend upon factors such as how competent you feel about dealing with the situation, the amount of support around you and the local *policies* and *procedures*.

Option 1

There are a number of methods which may be effective. Faced with an aggressive or violent person you should be aware of yourself first. Your body language and voice should be calm and non-threatening and you should not invade the person's personal space. Retain an open non-aggressive stance. Think about the way you are responding to the person and how you speak to them. Do not allow the person to think that you are going to take direct aggressive action against them or they will feel threatened.

You should never threaten or challenge the person, or defend situations/people that the person is feeling angry about. Do not ridicule or belittle them, but show respect for them even if they are not showing it for themselves or for you. Accept the full verbal expression of angry feelings (swearing will not hurt you!) and whenever possible remove bystanders to prevent possible injury or an audience. Most important of all:

Don't take chances; don't get hurt; know your limitations.

Option 2

Go away and get help. Make sure you are aware of the local *policies* and *procedures* for getting help. Never feel that you didn't do your job properly for we all have limitations and unfamiliar situations to deal with. If you accept these *limitations* and seek help you are dealing with the situation in the most competent and professional way.

Restraint

Occasionally an incident will become so severe that it may be necessary to physically restrain the client. The DHSS guideline (1976) dictates that 'In all such circumstances the initiative for taking or directing action should rest with the most appropriately experienced senior professional present'.

As a care assistant the decision as to whether physical restraint should be used will not be yours; however, you may be involved in the actual restraint. General principles for restraint are laid down within the DHSS guidelines. You need to be familiar with the procedures which apply in your work situation.

After the incident

After an incident has occurred you may experience many forms of emotion. Many people feel upset or worried that they may have caused the problems; others may feel angry or tired. Whatever your *feelings* are about the situation it is important to recognize that it is a natural response and that these feelings should not be ignored.

Your workplace may or may not have a *de-briefing* policy. De-briefing is a structured time to spend with colleagues and/or senior staff sharing your experience or feelings. For those of you who do not have a structured facility it is important to talk about the experience. Other support groups may be available within your workplace. Take advantage of these facilities (Fig. 3.3).

- Talk to your colleagues
- Share experiences
- Talk to your manager
- Share feelings

Recording and reporting

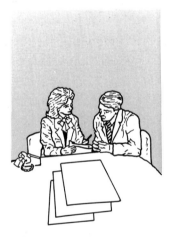

As soon after the incident as possible, a full and accurate report should be made to the appropriate person/s and entered into the *records*. Your department will have specifically designed forms for this purpose. The longer the period between the incident and the report, the more likely it is that the facts will become confused.

Important facts to record

- Name of person
- Description of difficult behaviour observed
- What happened immediately after the incident
- Length of incident
- What happened immediately before the incident
- Any other relevant information

Fig. 3.3 Take advantage of facilities to talk about experiences.

It is important to record and report each incident, whether a singular incident or regular occurrence. They are all of equal importance, as this will affect the care and treatment prescribed for the client and influence preventative actions to be taken against future outbursts.

Other reasons for recording and reporting are the need for good management and the need to ensure that any subsequent complaints can be dealt with. Ensure that all recording and reporting is made in a manner which maintains the client's confidentiality.

If you have been injured there will be additional procedures for you to follow and forms to be completed.

Activity 3.7 ■

 Find out: What procedure do you follow if you have been injured?

■ ■

Case study

> Maureen, a 44-year old woman, has arrived at your workplace for an appointment with your manager. Your manager has been called away for an urgent meeting and will not be able to see Maureen for another hour.
>
> Maureen appears upset on arrival and sits outside the manager's office. When you attempt to explain the delay Maureen becomes flushed, red in the face and starts to shake. She attempts to enter the manager's office, which is locked. When she realizes that the door is locked she begins hammering on the office door and screaming.

Activity 3.8 ■

 How would you attempt to deal with this situation? Try not to use Option 2 described earlier.

■ ■

There is no prescribed right answer, but by using the guidelines listed in the earlier section titled 'How do we deal with difficult behaviour?' you will hopefully be better equipped to defuse the situation effectively.

Summary

Now that you have worked through this chapter and completed Activities 3.1 to 3.8 you should have an increased awareness of yourself, others and the policies and procedures regarding difficult behaviour. Remember the key points:

(1) Don't take chances, don't get hurt
(2) Become aware of your limitations
(3) Read policies and procedures
(4) Prepare well
(5) Find out how to get help
(6) Keep updated

You may find it helpful to visit some areas to observe experts dealing with difficult behaviour every day. Once you have done this try looking at the activities in this chapter again. You may find that the answers you now give are quite different from your original ones.

References

Chamberlain, P. *STEP Manual*. The British Association of Behavioural Psychotherapy.

DHSS (1976) *The management of violent or potentially violent hospital patients.* DHSS Guideline H1 (76) 11. DHSS, London.

Further reading

Local organizational policies, procedures and guidelines.

The Code of Practice 1991

Finney, G. (1988) One false move. *Community Outlook*, April, 8–9.

Killen, S. (1983) Nurses and the mental health act. *Nursing Times*, 14 September, **79**(37), 46–8.

Leopold, H. (1985) The act translated … Mental Health Act 1983. *Nursing Times*, 16 October, **81**(42), 42–3.

Mason, P. (1991) Violent trends. *Nursing Times*, 22 May, **87**(21), 16–17.

Mental Health Act 1983. HMSO, London.

Miller, R. (1991) Hitting back. *Nursing Times*, 30 January, **87**(5), 56–8.

NUPE (1991) *Survey, Violence in the Health Service.* NUPE, London.

Smith, S. (1988) Take care, be aware … personal safety at work. *Community Outlook*, April, 10–12.

Whittington, R. (1989) Invisible injury. *Nursing Times*, 18 October, **85**(42), 30–32.

Whittington, R. & Wykes, T. (1989) Threatening behaviour. *Nursing Times*, 18 October, **85**(42), 26–9.

Wolf, F. (1991) Violence at work. *Living*, July, 22–5.

Wondrack, R. (1989) Dealing with verbal abuse. *Nurse Education Today*, **9**, 276–80.

Chapter 4
Obtaining and Storing Client Information
Rita Gale

Overview

One of the most important aspects of your work as a carer will involve you in the information which is included in the client's manual records or held on the computer system. It is vital to everyone concerned in delivering a care service to the client, and of course it is vital to the client as well, that these records are readily available, accurate and up-to-date.

As a carer you have direct contact with clients and therefore you are in the ideal position to obtain the appropriate information to ensure that clients' records are as comprehensive and up-to-date as possible. This chapter guides you through the ways in which you can obtain information, record and store it in manual records or on computer systems and the methods of retrieving it.

The rules of confidentiality are the same whatever the source of the information or the method by which it is recorded. This includes records held in GP practices and nursing records, such as plans of care, held in the client's home or a residential home. Every client has the absolute right to expect confidentiality to be maintained at all times.

Key words

Confidentiality, computer, information, log out, password, log in, medical records library, manual records, patient master index, tracking systems, menu, help facilities.

Confidentiality

As a carer, you will be responsible for maintaining at all times your organization's policy on *confidentiality*. You should therefore ask to see a copy of your organization's procedures on confidentiality to ensure that you, and others, observe the rules.

There are three Acts of Parliament of which you should be particularly aware, although you will never personally be authorized to release information in response to requests made under these Acts. Such requests can only be dealt with by a consultant or a senior manager from the administrative and clerical staff.

Data Protection Act 1984

This Act lays down strict guidelines on confidentiality and carries severe penalties for any breach of these. It includes allowing patients access to health records kept on *computer*, although certain *information* is exempt by virtue of the Subject Access Modification Order 1987.

Access to Medical Reports Act 1988

This Act covers requests from employers or insurance companies seeking medical reports on clients. For example, an employer or insurance company cannot seek a medical report for employment or insurance purposes, from the clinician responsible for the client's case, without the client's knowledge and consent. The client also has the right to see the report before it is passed to the employer/insurance company, to request that corrections be made and to refuse permission for the report to be released.

Access to Health Records Act 1990

This Act gives individuals the right of access, subject to certain exemptions, to health information about themselves recorded from 1 November 1991, other than on a *computer*, namely *manual records*. (Health records kept on computer are already accessible to the patient by virtue of section 21 of the Data Protection Act 1984 as modified by the Subject Access Modification Order 1987.)

Requests for information may be made directly by the client to the clinician, for example at an out-patient consultation, but otherwise all requests must be made in writing. Written requests are dealt with by a member of the administrative and clerical staff, who will seek permission from the appropriate clinician to release the information and also determine whether a fee should be charged to the client.

Disclosing information

Any requests you receive in person, by telephone or in writing, to disclose information held on computer or in manual records, should always be referred to your immediate manager. Never make the decision yourself as to what is, or is not, disclosable information.

Avoiding breaches of confidentiality

The relationship between the client and medical and nursing staff is based entirely on trust. It is essential both to the physical and mental well-being of the client that this trust is maintained at all times by strict observance of the rules of confidentiality.

The most common ways in which confidentiality can be breached are as follows:

- Notes left in an unattended area
- Failure to establish whether information may be disclosed
- Discussions about clients in public places
- Failure to *log out* of the computer system, allowing others access on your *password*

- Information on a VDU screen which is visible to the public
- Failure to establish a person's identity before disclosing information
- Allowing your password to be known and used by others
- Conducting conversations (including on the telephone) in a public area

Every member of staff is responsible for confidentiality within their organization. Therefore, if you observe the rules being breached you should inform the appropriate person.

Confidentiality and computer systems

Access levels

Access levels are a means of controlling which individuals have access to particular types of information on the computer system. You will be given a password appropriate to your needs for carrying out your duties. For example, you may need to access the bed-states function, but not the out-patients appointments system. You may also need, in certain circumstances, to input or amend information, whereas on other occasions you will only need to obtain information. The password you will be given will reflect your individual need.

It is essential that you never divulge your password to another person and that when you have finished using the system, you *log out* before leaving the terminal. This will prevent another person accessing the system using your *password*.

Siting of terminals

Terminals must always be sited with the screens facing away from public areas, so that the information can only be seen by the user (Fig. 4.1). Never walk away from the terminal leaving information visible on the screen. However short your absence, if you are called away whilst using the system, always log out and log in again on your return.

Fig. 4.1 Site a screen facing away from a public area.

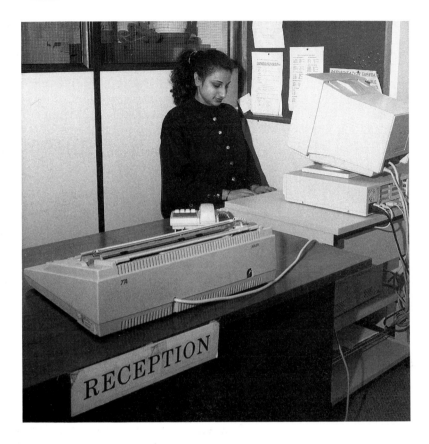

Tracking systems

Tracking is used on computer systems for the same purpose as tracer cards in manual systems. By accessing the client's details on the computer system, the tracking field will tell you the present location of the records.

With both tracer cards and tracking systems, however, the accuracy of the information reflects whether or not staff retrieving records from the library have updated the details on the manual or computer systems.

Confidentiality and access to libraries

As the library is an area containing highly confidential information, *access* to the library is usually strictly controlled. If you are not personally allowed to enter the library, you will find that medical records library staff will be available to retrieve records, or print microfilm, on request.

Medical records library

Clients' *manual medical records* (usually referred to as *Notes*) are stored and filed numerically in the *Medical Records Library*. Every client who attends an out-patient clinic or is admitted to a ward is registered on the *patient master index* and given a unique hospital number. This number is recorded on the computer system and on the front cover of the manual records file.

On each occasion that the client attends an out-patient clinic, or is admitted, the manual records will be required by the clinicians and will be *retrieved* from the medical library for that purpose. When the in-patient or out-patient episode is complete, the manual records are returned to the library for storing until they are required for another episode.

Microfilming of manual records (notes)

Because libraries do not have a limitless capacity for the storage of manual records, it is usual to *microfilm* selected sets of old records, which releases space for current records. The film spools on which information from the manual records is held are similar to the ones used in cameras. It is very easy to obtain copies of the required film by feeding the spool through a printing machine, identifying the appropriate documents and instructing the machine to print copies.

Tracer cards

Tracer cards are used in manual storage systems as a means of tracing the whereabouts of a set of records. When records are retrieved from the library, a tracer card must be completed and placed in the space left by removal of the file. The tracer card will state the date on which the file was retrieved, the clinic or ward involved and the name of the person borrowing the file. This information allows anyone else seeking the records to identify when, and by whom, the file was retrieved from the library (Fig. 4.2).

Retrieving records from other hospitals

When you need to obtain records from another hospital, it is usual for such requests to go through the medical records library. The library will contact the hospital concerned and arrange for the transportation of the records by the fastest and safest route. As this process can take a few days, it is prudent to give the medical records library as much advance notice as possible.

Obtaining information about a client

The main sources of information about a client are as follows:

Fig. 4.2 Retrieving
records from the library.

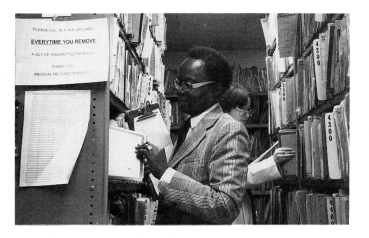

(1) General practitioner referral letter.
(2) Patient questionnaire (which is usually sent to each client with the first out-patient appointment).
(3) Direct from the client at an out-patient clinic attendance.
(4) Information already in the client's notes.
(5) The admissions office (for in- patients).
(6) Direct from the client, or the client's relatives, during an in-patient episode.
(7) Colleagues on duty at the time of the admission.
(8) Computer systems.

The means of obtaining information falls into three categories:

■ Face-to-face interviews   ■ Written information
■ Telephone

Face-to-face interviews

By this method you receive the information direct from the source concerned. This makes sure that the information is accurate, and gives you the chance to resolve any queries on the spot.

It is sometimes necessary to ask a client for information of a sensitive nature, which may cause them some distress. This problem can usually be overcome by explaining carefully why the information is needed. If you have reason to believe that a question may be particularly sensitive, it is helpful to explain first why you need the information. Clients will usually appreciate and respond favourably to questions asked in a sensitive manner.

Face-to-face interviews for the purpose of obtaining information should always be conducted with regard to a client's right to privacy.

Written information

Written information should be *legible*, *accurate* and *concise*. A brief heading identifying the subject contained in the message immediately informs the reader of the type of information the writer is going to convey. For example, if the heading reads 'Urology clinic – booking of appointments' the writer has in just five words identified which clinic is being referred to and which activity within that clinic.

Written information should always include the names of the *sender* and *recipient*, the date, the time (when a message is received by telephone), the department or location and, if appropriate, the telephone number. These details enable sender and recipient to contact each other without delay should the need arise.

Telephone

This is a commonly used way to obtain information, but is also one where misunderstandings and errors can easily occur. Many of these errors are caused by the speaker failing to communicate in an *articulate* manner, which in turn can lead to confusion and misunderstanding.

The following guidelines will help you to avoid the common pitfalls of obtaining information through the medium of the telephone:

(1) Identify yourself to the recipient of the call.
(2) Confirm you have the correct department or location.
(3) State briefly the reason for the call, for example 'This is the admissions office with a query on your bed state'.
(4) Deliver the message as concisely as possible and, if appropriate, in the correct sequence of events.
(5) Ask the recipient to repeat back to you any details you feel it might be prudent to confirm, for example 'There are eight empty beds on the ward at present'.
(6) Make a brief written record of the conversation, including the name of the person with whom you spoke, the date and time of the call and what action, if any, was taken as a result.

Information from computer systems

The patient information provided by the computer will only be as accurate and complete as the data input to the system. Extreme care and attention to detail at the time of obtaining information, by whatever method, is therefore essential.

Recording information in manual records

Entering information in a client's records for both clinical and non- clinical purposes requires legible handwriting and the use of good basic English.

This prevents any confusion arising from an erroneous interpretation of illegible handwriting or misunderstanding of unfamiliar words.

The file containing the manual records usually has an *index insert* to indicate, for example, the section in which documentation referring to out-patient attendances is filed. There will also be a *mount sheet* for test results from, say, the haematology department, and a separate one for X-ray department results.

Correspondence should always be *secured* inside the file in the appropriate section and test results fixed to the correct mount sheet, with nothing left loose in the file. If these procedures are followed, anyone wishing to obtain information from the manual records can do so easily and without delay.

Every entry which you make in the manual records should state the date and time at which you wrote the information and your name or initials.

Inputting information on computer systems

The data which you input will probably be accessed by many other members of staff and therefore it is essential that you check the accuracy of the information before *inputting* to the computer system.

Many of the client's details, such as address and date of birth, will have been input at the time of registration. You may, however, sometimes find it necessary to input additional information or *amend* some of the details if, for example, the client has changed an address or telephone number.

If you are inputting information from a written form or patient questionnaire, it is prudent to check the date on which the client provided the information. If some considerable time has elapsed between this date and actual input some of the details might be out of date. It is for this reason that clients should be asked at each out-patient attendance, or in-patient episode, whether there is any change to their basic details.

Menu

The *menu* lists all the functions available on the module. Against each function, for example waiting lists, there will be a code which, when entered, will give you access to the information, provided your password allows you entry.

'Help' facility

Computer programs are usually written in such a way as to provide prompts or *help* facilities in appropriate fields, particularly *mandatory* ones. For example, if you select the help facility in the field of requesting the client's religion, the screen will display a number of options from which you can select the appropriate religion.

Computer systems are widely used sources of information, which can only be as comprehensive and accurate as the users inputting the data allow them to be.

Patient master index

The patient master index is the most frequently accessed function on the computer system and holds the following details:

Hospital number:
Surname:
Forename:
Title:
Date of birth:
Address (including postcode):
Marital status:
General practitioner:
Sex:

The information held on the patient master index allows for the accurate collection of information and statistics, by the Department of Health, on a national basis.

The patient data required by the Department of Health are increasingly being extended, with the result that computer programs frequently have to be upgraded to meet the need for recording additional information. Most organizations employ staff for the specific purpose of registering clients on the patient master index, but you may on occasion need to amend information held on the system. It is essential that updated information is entered on to the system without delay. For example, failure to update a client's telephone number could mean that the client could not be contacted if a bed became available at short notice, or if a test result indicated that an urgent out-patient attendance was required.

Fig. 4.3 Collecting information from new clients.

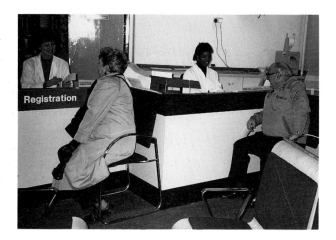

Charges for treatment

Treatment automatically exempt from charges

Automatic exemption applies to all treatment given in the following departments:

- Accident and emergency
- Dental emergency
- Ophthalmic emergency

This exemption extends to all clients, whether residents of the UK or visitors to this country, who require emergency treatment. Clients suffering from a notifiable infectious disease are always exempt from NHS charges, whatever their status. It should be noted that for clients diagnosed as being HIV/AIDS positive, the automatic exemption is restricted to diagnostic tests and counselling only. If treatment is then required, the status of the client must be established.

Identifying overseas visitors

All clients attending an NHS hospital must be assessed to determine whether they are exempt from charges for treatment. This assessment applies equally to clients resident in the UK and to those from overseas countries.

At a client's first attendance at the out-patient clinic, or on admittance to a ward that is not the result of an out-patient appointment (for example the accident and emergency department), they will be asked the question 'Have you been resident in the UK for the past 12 months?'. It should be noted that the UK consists of the following:

- England (not including the Channel Islands and the Isle of Man)
- Scotland
- Wales
- Northern Ireland (not Eire)

The majority of clients will answer 'yes' to this question and are therefore exempt from charges. However, if the client answers 'no' then it will be necessary for the client's status to be investigated further. These investigations can be quite complex and, in most organizations, are carried out by specially trained members of staff.

As a carer, your role in identifying overseas visitors will usually be limited to checking that the status of the client has been established and that the information has been recorded, either on the computer system or in the manual records. It is essential that clients who are not eligible to receive free NHS treatment pay the appropriate health authority for the cost of their treatment.

Summary

All information concerning clients is held either in manual medical records or on the computer system. As a carer, you will be one of the staff responsible for obtaining, inputting and updating this confidential information.

In both manual and computer systems there is a great need for accuracy. This is as important for recording telephone numbers as it is for recording clinical details. Users of both systems depend upon each other for the record they see to be both accurate and up-to-date.

When not in current use, manual records must always be stored in the medical records library. The outer file must be in good condition and the documentation securely fastened inside.

Computer screens must never be visible to the public, and preferably only to the user. Always remember to log out of the system when you have finished accessing the information.

Confidentiality must be maintained at all times, together with respect for the privacy and dignity of the client.

Further reading

Organizational policies and procedures concerning confidentiality and patients' records.

Data Protection Act 1984

Access to Health Records Act 1991

Vousden, M. (1987) Do you really need to know? *Nursing Times*, **83**(49), 28–30.

Chapter 5
Mobility and Safer Client Handling
Fay Reid

Overview

There is very little nursing care that is undertaken for or with a client that does not involve moving them. If we are going to assist clients with their daily activities then we need to become competent in moving them. To develop this skill you will need to watch demonstrations by expert practitioners and then practise for yourselves. Very few of us learn to drive a car or play a musical instrument without practice. This chapter will give you some guidance and serve to reinforce what you have been shown.

Key words

Legal responsibilities, care plan, mobility assessment, space, equipment, safe systems, synchronization.

Caring for clients with mobility problems

We all need to move. We need to move to find, prepare and eat food. We move as quickly as we can to get away from danger. We wriggle to make ourselves comfortable and to even out the pressures on our body when we are sitting or lying. There are however some people, who, either because of disease or physical frailty, cannot do this for themselves and will need you to help them.

The task of moving people is not an easy one as they are almost always longer, heavier or larger than you think. They do not have handles, or grab-slots. They can be stiffer or floppier than you imagine and have arms and legs that wave about and do not always do what they should, or stay where you have placed them. They can be unstable and unbalanced and behave in an apparently irrational manner.

Check the client's care plan

Before you attempt to move clients always check with the *care plan*, which will have been completed following the assessment of the client. You need to know how much and what the clients can do for themselves so that you can encourage them to do it. Clients have a right to independence, to continue to do for themselves those activities that they can manage. We should not condition clients into dependence because we find it quicker to do something for them rather than allowing them to do it for themselves. The care plan should give you information on what the client can manage, what technique to use and how many carers may be needed. It should also give you information on the *client handling equipment* that is considered necessary in order to move the client *safely*.

Familiarize yourself with the equipment

Make friends with the client handling equipment. It has been provided to enable you to move clients as comfortably and as safely as possible for both yourself and the client. To acquire a painful back because you moved a client who was too heavy for you is not helpful for either your colleagues, your clients or yourself.

Legislation relating to safety at work

According to the Health and Safety at Work etc. Act 1974 in Chapter 37, Part 1, section 2, sub-sections (a) to (e):

- Your employer is required to provide and maintain *equipment* and *safe systems* of work.
- Your employer is also required to give you information, instruction and supervision.
- Transport and storage of equipment must be safe and there must be ease of access to and from wherever you are working.
- You must co-operate with your employer in the safe use of equipment which is provided and take the opportunities that you are given in relation to training.

As you can see the Act contains *responsibilities* for both yourself and your employer.

There are two more Acts of Parliament that you need to know about. The first is the Reporting of Injuries, Diseases and Dangerous Occurrences Regulations 197, 1985, known as RIDDOR for short. This requires a senior manager to make a report to the regional office of the Health and Safety Executive of any accident that has resulted in more than three days off work. You will find that the majority of incident/accident reporting forms have a small insert at the bottom corner asking if the incident requires a report on form F2508, the official form. It is very important that incidents are reported so that the statistics are as accurate as possible and also to allow managers to identify those areas where staff are at a particular risk.

Activity 5.1 ■■■■■■■■■■■■■■■■■■■■■■■■■■■■■

 Look in your workplace for your accident/incident forms for recording all incidents.

■■■■■■■■■■■■■■■■■■■■■■■■■■■■■■■■■■■■

The third place of legislation is an EC Directive that required national governments that are signatories to the directive, including the UK, to implement their own legislation by 1 January 1993. The Manual Handling of Operations Regulations 1992 require all employers to make an assessment of the task if there is any risk of back injury in the load handling task. The regulations define handling as pushing, pulling, lifting, lowering, supporting or moving by hand or bodily force. A load is defined as a discrete movable object and includes human beings and animals. The Royal College of Nursing has produced a Code of Practice for client handling that reflects the guidelines of the Manual Handling of Operations Regulations 1992.

Activity 5.2 ■■■■■■■■■■■■■■■■■■■■■■■■■■■■■

 Make yourself familiar with your local policies and guidelines concerning safe manual handling. These should be available in your workplace and are based on the Health and Safety at Work etc. Act 1974.

■■■■■■■■■■■■■■■■■■■■■■■■■■■■■■■■■■■■

Principles of safe lifting

To acquire a skill requires knowledge and practice. Nurse teachers or physiotherapists will demonstrate *safe client handling techniques* and provide you with the opportunities to practise and to develop your skills – you need to make the most of them. This chapter is a little like a recipe book; it can tell you what to do but you cannot claim that you *know how* to do it until you see a technique demonstrated and have practised it a number of times.

Some of the principles will be examined in more detail:

■ *Get as close to the load as you can.*

Activity 5.3 ■■■■■■■■■■■■■■■■■■■■■■■■■■■■

 Try this little experiment. Pile two large heavy books on top of each other, or use something that weighs about 3 kg (approximately 7 lb). Hold it close to you and think how you feel. Now hold it away from you and feel the difference. The load is just the same and you are the same but it seems much harder. You haven't grown weaker; it takes more effort because the load is further away from you.

■■■■■■■■■■■■■■■■■■■■■■■■■■■■■■■■■■■■

■ *Always keep your back straight and your head up.*

Activity 5.4 ■

To find out what stooping does to you, stand as comfortably as possible then lean your body forward until you are 20° out of the vertical. Hold that position for a minute and a half and try to remember what your muscles tell you while you are standing like that.

■ ■

Activity 5.5 ■

One day, when you are at home, or at work, try recording the amount of time that you spend in a stooped position. You may be surprised.

■ ■

■ *Make sure you have a good wide base.* Stand with one foot forward so that the load is positioned between your feet and one foot is flat on the floor. Avoid bending so that your heels are off the floor as you will be unstable.

■ *Bend your knees and use your strong thigh muscles to push* yourself to a standing position.

■ *Avoid twisting*, particularly if you are picking something up or carrying it. Use your feet to cut down the stress on your back by pivoting. Aim to keep your hips and shoulders in alignment.

■ Use the command '*ready, steady, lift*' when you are lifting with another or several carers. This is much clearer than 'one, two, three lift'. When carers use 'one, two, three', one person always lifts early and another lifts late and someone gets hurt.

Holding the client

Use a wide, open, relaxed hand to hold the client if you are guiding or assisting them to move. A tense hand hold may convey nervousness or anxiety to the client, who may in turn react by becoming tense as well.

Activity 5.6 ■

To experience the effect of tension on yourself, sit on a chair, preferably one with arms, so that you can rest your own arms on them. Relax your left arm so that it is resting comfortably. Now clench your right fist as hard as you possibly can and hold it for a minute or two. When the time is up unclench your hand and think how it feels. Do your fingers want to open wide or close up again? If you feel tension in your hand just think what it does to you if your body is continually tense.

■ ■

When you are moving a client *always* explain what you are going to do and seek the client's cooperation. You may find it helpful to ask the client to take a deep breath in when you say 'steady' and to breathe out when you say 'lift' or 'up' or whatever activity you are carrying out.

Grips used with another carer

There are a number of grips that can be used when you are working with another carer. There are advantages and disadvantages for each grip which will be discussed.

Activity 5.7 ■

Practise these grips with a colleague. Remember when you do so that you will be working on opposite sides of the bed and you need to be moving in the same direction.

■ ■

Finger grip

The carers grasp each other's hands, locking fingers together. This gives extra length to the grip which can be useful. However if your fingernails are longer than the pulp of your fingers then it could be so painful for your colleague that she loosens her grip and leaves you holding the full weight of the client.

Single wrist grip

One carer holds the wrist of the second carer. The free hand of the second carer can be used to give a feeling of extra security to the client by using a relaxed palm hold on them.

Double wrist grip

Each carer holds the wrist of the other. Some people find that this puts considerable strain on their wrists. This is a very strong grip. It can also be used as a double fore-arm or elbow grip.

Moving a client's limbs

If you are asked to hold or move a client's limb, remember to hold the arm or leg above and below a joint. To pick arms and legs up and hold them in the air by toes or fingers is painful for the client and could be harmful for you. Legs can be very heavy and it is not easy to get close to lift them. Slide your hands under the limb, and bend your knees so that you can maintain a straight back. Have one foot a step ahead of the other and get close to the bed, chair or whatever the client is on. It is sometimes helpful to rest the client's foot or hand on your shoulder.

Sitting the client up

Many clients need to be sat up; they slide down the bed and need to sit up to aid their breathing. To hold them under the armpits and pull them into a sitting position is painful for them and dangerous for you. If the client can manage it, get them to bend their knees with their feet flat on the bed; then encourage them to roll gently to the side and push up with their hands. This method takes away the strain from the abdomen.

Activity 5.8 ■

 Try this method of sitting yourself up when you are lying in bed. It is safer for you than sitting straight up.

■ ■

If clients cannot sit up by themselves then take either a handling sling or the client's own towel folded lengthways into three and position this carefully behind their shoulders. This gives greater leverage and allows you to pull the client into a sitting position without damage to yourself or the client. If the client is stiff or heavy you will need someone on the other side of the client to help. You will also need someone to support the client while you re-arrange pillows, etc.

Moving a client up the bed

You may find, having sat the client up, that there is a gap between the client and the pillows. Even if there are two of you, resist the temptation to pick the client up and carry them up the bed. Sometimes the client will be able to move on their own using either a monkey pole or hand blocks.

Moving oneself up the bed is quite an awkward manoeuvre. The weight of the body causes the mattress to sink and our arms are not long enough to lift the trunk clear of the mattress. It is essential that the buttocks are raised well clear of the bed as any dragging can cause friction, which may result in tissue damage and a possible pressure sore. Hand blocks are very useful in these circumstances as they add length to the arms, enabling the trunk to be raised and eased backwards. Monkey poles can also be used to help clients to move themselves, but it requires more shoulder girdle strength to pull oneself up than it does to push up. Women are usually less likely than men to use a monkey pole effectively as, generally, their shoulder muscles are not as well developed.

Australian/shoulder lift

This is one of the safest lifts as it is less likely to raise intra-abdominal pressure of the carer to potentially damaging levels. It should only be used on clients weighing less than 8 stone (112 lb or 51 kg) who are being nursed on variable height beds.

In order to get close to the load you need to face the direction of the lift and put the knee that is closer to the bed on the bed parallel with the client's thighs. Your knee should be level with the client's back.

The shoulder that is next to the client is placed in the client's axilla (armpit) and that hand grasps your partner's wrist or fore-arm under the client's thighs, well above the knees. You may find it helpful to use a client handling sling under the client's thighs. This gives greater support to the client and gives you a firm grip with a variable distance.

The hand that is further from the client is placed on the mattress to brace your trunk and give support. The client's arms are placed down your back in a position that is comfortable for both of you.

Before starting this lift you must discuss who will give the command to lift and which hand or wrist grip will be used. The command that you should use is 'Ready, steady, lift'.

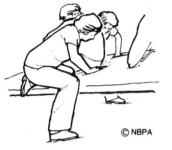

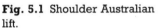

Fig. 5.1 Shoulder Australian lift.

Turning a client in bed

There are many reasons for turning a client in bed. It could be to change their position, or a sheet, wash their back or check their pressure areas, and there are a number of ways of doing it. The client's condition will dictate the correct method and ideally it should be recorded in the care plans.

If the client is in the centre of the bed and you need to turn them on to their side then, providing there is no contra-indication, simply ask them to bend their knees and roll them towards the side of the bed. This manoeuvre has the client halfway towards you.

Then place your knee on the bed – this helps to prevent the client from rolling out of the bed. Take the client's hand which is furthest from you into whichever of your hands is nearest the foot of the bed. Pull very gently and the client will roll towards you. Put your foot back on the floor. This technique can also be used as the start of taking a client out of bed.

The easiest method to relieve pressure is to use the 30° tilt. It allows the client to be eased from soft tissue to soft tissue and avoids pressure on the bony prominences. It is more comfortable for the patient and less tiring for the carer. The bottom sheet is used to turn the client and pillows are used to maintain the position.

Standing at the side of the bed, hold the sheet from the opposite side at the client's shoulder and hip and pull it towards yourself. If the client is very heavy two people may be needed, but often one is enough. Pulling the sheet will cause the client to roll towards you. When the client's body is at an angle of about 40° off the bed your colleague can ease the pillows under the client's back and the client will then relax back against them, maintaining an angle of approximately 30°. The sheet can then be tucked back under the mattress.

When the client needs to be moved again a further 30° tilt can be undertaken, bringing the client's body to an angle of 60°. Alternatively a 30° tilt can be made to the opposite side.

If the client is already on their side and you need to turn them to the opposite side, remove the packing or pillows that are supporting them and guide them gently on to their back. The safest way to undertake this task is to use either a Rotaprone, an Easy-glide or an Easy-slide. If you do not have these items then you may have to turn the client manually. Remember, if the client weighs more than 8 stone (112 lb or 51 kg) they should be turned using a non-manual technique.

Ideally there should be at least two of you to complete this task. Use the natural hollows of the body and try to apportion the weight of the client's body equally. This may be best achieved by one of you taking neck to waist and the other taking waist to under thighs. In this way the weight of the trunk is more evenly divided. Slide your hands into the hollows, taking care not to trap the client's skin. Give the order and draw the client gently towards you into the middle of the bed. The client is then ready to be turned on to their opposite side.

The following method of moving a client on your own should be done with the greatest of care and only if they are light. With the client on their back move the legs towards you; then lift the head and shoulders; finally slide your hands under the client and draw the buttocks towards you. You can then turn them on to their side.

Standing the client up

Ensure that you know exactly what the client is capable of doing. If the client is on a rehabilitation programme and the physiotherapist has shown a way of standing, try to use the same technique to avoid confusing the client.

Activity 5.9 ■

 Think what you do when you stand up. You wriggle to the front of the chair, place your feet flat on the floor, then using the arms of the chair you push forward into a *nose over toes* position and push up.

■ ■

You do the same thing with a client. If the client cannot wriggle themselves to the front of the chair you will need to help them. Stand in front of them with bent knees and, using a relaxed palm hold in a *cup a bum* grip, you bring each buttock forward in turn until the client is in the correct position to lean forward and put their *nose over their toes*. Encourage the client to grasp the arms of the chair and push themselves up.

For some patients who have had a stroke and whose quadriceps (thigh muscles) are still strong on the unaffected side, another way is occasionally used. It starts the same way as the first method until the *nose over toes* position is reached, then the client is encouraged to swing their arms to help get *lift off*.

Stand on the weaker side of the client to help to bring the weaker hip forward. This enables the client to come to a balanced standing position instead of putting all their weight through the unaffected leg. If they cannot do this for themselves then you can assist them. The client holds you round the waist (a belt gives him something to hold on to). If he cannot reach with both arms then he can place one hand on your shoulder.

Never allow the client to clasp you around the neck. Should the client fall or go into an extensor spasm while clasping you around the neck their weight would be suspended on your cervical spine and you could sustain a very severe neck injury.

If the client is wearing a belt that you can hold on to, use it. If not, a client handling sling will give you a more stable grip. Rock the client backwards and forwards until they start to leave the chair seat, then lever them up to a standing position.

When the client needs two people to stand them up, then providing that they can bear weight you can use either a SARA (standing and raising aid) if you have one, or the human equivalent. Facing the back of the chair you put your shoulder into the client's axilla and that hand holds the client's waist on the opposite side. Your partner does the same. The client's arms and hands are placed down your back as in the Australian/shoulder lift. Your free hand is used to brace yourself on the arm of the chair. The command 'ready, steady, stand' is given and both carers stand up. The client is supported by both carers' arms and hands, and feels very safe (Fig. 5.2).

Walking the client

Before you walk a client you need to ensure that they are able to do what you are asking them to do. If you are trying to walk the client to a lavatory that is 12 metres from where they are sitting and they can only walk 2 metres you will have a problem when they can go no further. If they are using an aid such as a walking stick, frame or crutches (Fig. 5.3), check that the rubber ferrule still has its pattern on it and that it hasn't worn smooth. Make sure that it is the correct height for the client.

Stand on the weaker side of the client using a palm to palm thumb grip. You should be holding the client's right hand with your right hand or their left hand with your left hand. This allows the hand that is nearest the client

Fig. 5.2 Assisting a
client to stand.

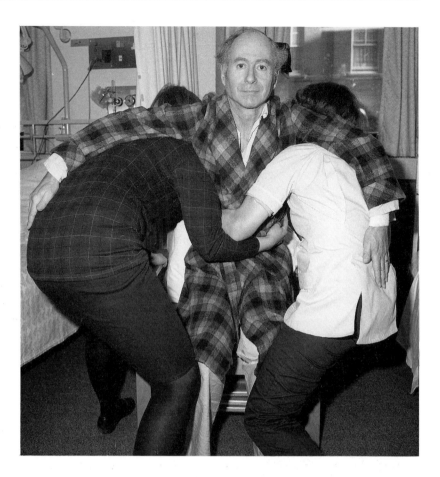

to be placed around the client's waist. This gives you control of the situation
should the client feel faint or fall. You need to walk very close to and slightly
behind the client so that you can take appropriate action very quickly.

Never attempt to catch the falling client and hold them up. The aim is
to break the client's fall so that their head does not strike the floor. This
technique is also aimed at preventing you from acquiring a very painful
injury.

Controlling a fall

In order for you to become skilled at this technique it should be demonstrated by experienced practitioners and practised under supervision. If you
feel the client start to sag let go of their hand and waist and move behind
them, putting one leg forward with a bent knee. Put your arms under the
client's axillae (armpits) until the client is resting in the crook of your
elbows. At the same time pull the client back against you to stabilize them

as you rest them on your thigh. At this point lower your arms and slide or guide your client to the floor.

Sitting a client in a chair

When positioning a client in a chair ensure that they are sitting with their back against the chair back so that they are well supported. If the chair does not support the client's head, they may find it comfortable to have a small pillow tucked behind their head. The chair back should be sufficiently comfortable so that a pillow is not needed behind the client. A pillow behind the client's back will eventually push them forward and you will then need to move them back into the chair.

The client's feet should be flat on the floor just about hip distance apart; this gives a more stable base. Try to ensure that the lower third of the client's thighs are not in contact with the chair. To sit comfortably there should be no pressure under the lower third of the thighs, otherwise there is a tendency to wriggle forward to relieve it. We sit more comfortably if only the upper third of the thigh is in contact with the chair. If the chair seat is high or if the client is short a low foot stool can be used to raise the client's legs and to take the pressure off the thighs.

Moving a client back in a chair

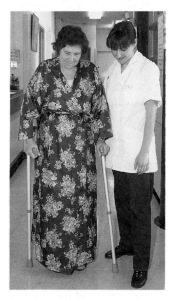

Fig. 5.3 Client with physiotherapist and using crutches.

After sitting for a while some clients manage to slide to the edge of the chair. *On no account should you lean over the back of the chair and attempt to pull the client back up.* That would put enormous strain on your back and it is not an efficient way to move them as you are simply pulling them into the chair back. Ensure that their buttocks are still on the chair. If they are not, place several pillows on the floor and lower the client on to them. The client can then be picked up using a *hoist*. It would be very dangerous to attempt to lift the client back on to the chair if they already have their buttocks off it.

If their buttocks are still on the chair then you can use the following technique to sit them back into it. Help the client to sit forward, i.e. in a *nose over toes* position. You can do this either with a relaxed palm grip, pulling them forward, or by using a client handling sling or folded towel. Get the client to hold you around your waist and use a handling sling around their buttocks. Pull the client gently forward, and their buttocks will leave the seat of the chair. Block the client's feet with your feet and place your knees against theirs. As the client's buttocks slightly lift from the chair, use your body weight to push against their knees. Your weight will push the client back into the chair.

Pivot transfers

These can be through either 90°, as when you are taking a client off their bed to put them into a chair, or 180°, if you need to put a client on to a lavatory from a wheelchair when there is restricted access and the client has to be turned to face the opposite direction.

The safest way to carry out this manoeuvre, if the client can bear weight, is with a hoist, in particular a SARA.

A turntable is another simple but effective tool that can be used, but again the client must have trunk stability and be able to weight bear. Put the brakes on the wheelchair, place the client's feet on the turntable and use either a belt to hold the client or a handling sling. Rock the client to a standing position then turn them and sit them down again.

If you haven't got a turntable or a hoist then you need to move the client's feet so that they do not get in the way. If you are going to turn the client from their left side towards their right side then place their left foot in front of and slightly across the right foot. If you are turning from right to left then the right foot goes in front of the left foot.

Trolley to bed or bed to trolley transfers

These transfers are very common. Clients go to the X-ray or the operating department and they have to be moved from their bed on to a trolley, often when they have been given pre-medication. They also have to be transferred back into their bed from a trolley when they may still be under the influence of the anaesthetic.

Sliding transfers are the safest way of doing this. There are a number of sliding transfer systems and they all have their advantages and disadvantages. One of the most comfortable from the client's point of view is the *Easy- slide*. This is a Norwegian invention and is like an open-ended sleeping bag. The material on the inside is almost friction-free so it rolls on itself. The Easy-slide is tucked half under the client underneath a sheet. When the command is given, one nurse pushes and the other on the far side of the trolley pulls. The client slides over quite effortlessly and comfortably (Fig. 5.4). The Pat-slide and Easy-glide work on similar principles, but they are firm boards and not quite so comfortable.

Note that *poles and canvas transfers are potentially dangerous* as the client's weight is a long way from the carer. Even with one person holding each pole there is still the danger of an unsynchronized lift. Furthermore, the carers standing furthest from the bed may well complete the lift holding the client's weight with their own backs twisted and bent and with their arms at full stretch.

Hoists

The use of a hoist should be planned into patient care and not due to an after thought or an emergency situation. There are a wide range of hoists

Fig. 5.4 Transferring a client using the Easy-slide.

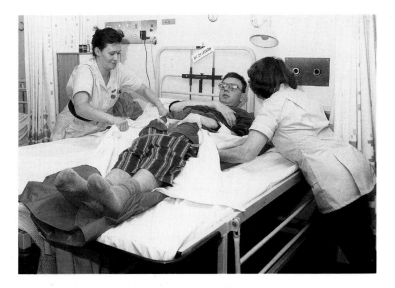

on the market and each tends to have its own function. There are relatively few hoists that will undertake a range of tasks and usually when they do it is something of a compromise.

Activity 5.10 ■

 Look for the hoist in your ward. What make is it? What task does it perform? What weight of client will it support? Is it fixed, mobile or ceiling mounted? Is it electrically, battery or manually operated? Is the mast tall enough to allow you to put the patient back on to a low air loss or Clinitron fluidized bed? Are the manufacturer's instructions available to you, either with the hoist or somewhere immediately accessible for you to read? Does the ward have a training programme?

■ ■

When using a hoist you should always use the slings designed for that model. If you use incorrect slings the manufacturers will not accept liability if there is an accident.

Activity 5.11 ■

 Find the slings that are used with the hoist on the ward. Are they colour coded for size? Colour coding makes it easy to identify the size of the sling and on some hoists guidance is given in relation to the weight it will hold. What weight will the hoists in your clinical area support?

■ ■

When placing slings on a client make sure that the seams face outward as they can be quite rough, particularly for clients with sensitive skins.

Fig. 5.5 Patient hoist handling.

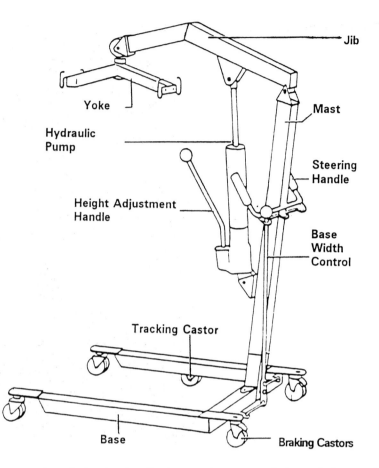

Never push a hoist by its jib, it may become unbalanced. It is only necessary to raise the client high enough to clear the bed easily. Once the sling has been placed around or under the client, lower the bed to its lowest level. It is then easier to raise the patient. As the height of the lift is dependent on the length of the mast, when the bed is high there is less height available. This may not be a problem if the client is short, but if the client is tall then a high bed will not allow you to raise the client off the bed.

Slings

The majority of slings are C- shaped. The legs of the C may be longer in some slings than others and the nylon straps that are used to secure the sling on the hoist may be of different lengths. Most slings are made of nylon, but different fabrics are available, for example fleece and net. The original chains have been replaced by nylon straps, which are quieter and less worrying for the client. Some of you may find, in ward bathrooms, white plastic bands with chains which are the original slings. These are cold and uncomfortable and not recommended for use. Figure 5.6 illustrates the use of a hoist with a sling.

Fig. 5.6 Using a hoist with a sling.

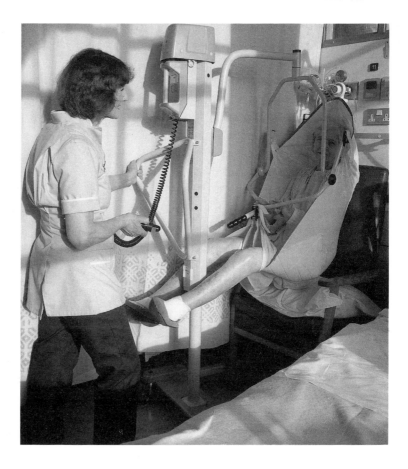

Bathing the client

Activity 5.12   ■

 Get into a dry bath and sit down. Now try to stand up without using your arms. You may be surprised to find how difficult it is. Pretend that you cannot use the arm and leg on the same side of your body and try to stand up again. Remember, while you are working out how, or if, you can stand, that the older we get the less muscle strength and tone we have. Finally try to get out of the bath using just your arms and not your legs.

■ ■

You will now have discovered the reason why we need *hoists* to take clients out of the bath – it is a very difficult handling task. Many of you will be familiar with the toilet chair and its removable sub-frame which enables you to put a client in, and more importantly take them out of, a bath.

There are many varieties of bath hoist on the market and you need to become familiar with the type that is in the bathroom. There are side-loading and end-loading bath hoists. You cannot use an end-loading bath when the bath is against a wall. A side-loading hoist can only be used if the legs can go under the bath.

Moving the client from the floor

There are a number of ways of raising the client who has fallen to the floor, depending on the situation. The first action to take is to call for assistance in order for injuries, potential and actual, to be identified and treated if necessary.

Do not rush to lift the client from the floor. Make them comfortable (an up-ended chair padded with pillows makes a very comfortable back-rest if the client can sit up) while the necessary help and equipment are found.

Sometimes, once the client has rested and had a cup of tea, they can get themselves up by using a chair:

(1)   The client bends their knees with feet flat on the floor and rolls to the side and continues the roll until they are on hands and knees.
(2)   Both hands are placed on the chair seat and using the chair seat as a support, one knee is brought up and the arm on the same side is placed on the back of the chair.
(3)   This sequence is repeated with the other side.

If the client is too heavy or dependent to do this then a *hoist* must be used. A general purpose sling is used; some practitioners prefer to use a slightly larger size of sling when the client is to be removed from the floor.

If you are in a situation where *no hoist* is available then it requires *six* people to take someone off the floor:

(1)   You will need a strong blanket, counterpane or sheet, which is rolled under the client.
(2)   Then the carers position themselves one at each corner of the blanket or sheet, etc., with another person at each side level with the client's hips.
(3)   Decide on which way the team will move.
(4)   Roll blanket up to give the handlers a firm grip.
(5)   The order 'ready, steady, lift' is given clearly.
(6)   The team walk to the bed or trolley and pass on either side to the head of it. This enables the client to be placed in the middle of the bed.

Summary

This chapter is only an introduction to the complex topic of mobility and handling the human load. You need to develop your level of knowledge by studying some of the books that have been suggested as further reading at the end of this chapter. To summarize:

(1)   Check with the care plan to identify your client's needs.
(2)   Know what your client can do.
(3)   Consider what requires to be done.
(4)   Plan what you are going to do.
(5)   Ensure that everyone knows what the plan is.
(6)   Give clear instructions.
(7)   Work together.
(8)   Keep the load as close as possible.
(9)   Keep your back straight and your head up.
(10)   Bend your knees and use your strong thigh muscles.

References

Health and Safety at Work Act 1974, Chapter 37, Part 1. HMSO, London.

Health and Safety Commission (1992) *Manual Handling of Operations 1992 – Regulations and Guidance.* HMSO, London.

RCN Advisory Panel for Back Pain in Nurses (1993) *Code of Practice for the Handling of Patients*, 3rd edn. Royal College of Nursing, London.

Further reading

Birnbaum, R., Cockcroft, C., Richardson, B. & Corlett, N. (1992) *Safer Handling of Loads at Work – a Practical Ergonomics Guide.* Institute of Ergonomics, University of Nottingham.

Buckley, N. (1991) How safe is your ward? *Nursing Times*, **87**(6), 32–33.

Hill, C. & Cowan, V. (1987) Lifting – where prevention is the only cure. *Occupational Health*, November, 349–63.

Hill, I. (1983) Equipment for the job. *Nursing Times*, 6 July, **79**(27), 24–7.

Hollis, M. (1991) *Safer Lifting for Patient Care*, 3rd edn. Blackwell Scientific Publications, Oxford.

Okunowo, R. (1992) Home truths. *Nursing Standard*, 29 April, **6**(32), 55.

Pheasant, S. & Stubbs, D. (1991) *Lifting and Handling – an Ergonomic Approach.* National Back Pain Association, Teddington.

Stubbs, D. (1986) *Epidemiology of Back Pain in Nurses.* Robens Institute, University of Surrey.

Stubbs, D. & Buckle, P. (1984) The epidemiology of back pain in nurses. *Nursing*, 2nd series, number 32, December (number 33 useful as well).

Tarling, C. (1980) *Hoists and their uses.* Heinemann, London.

Troup, J.D.G. & Edwards, F. (1985) *Manual Handling and Lifting.* HMSO, London.

Troup, J.D.G., Lloyd, P., Osbourne, C., Tarling, C. & Wright, B. (1992) *The Handling of Patients – a Guide for Nurses*, 3rd edn. National Back Pain Association, Teddington.

Walsh, R. (1988) On the move. *Human Kinetics*, 31 August, **84**(35), 26–30 (continued 7 and 14 September 1988).

Wright, B. (1992) Patient handling – getting it right. *Nursing Standard*, 29 April, **6**(32), 52–3.

Chapter 6
Control of Infection
Heather Rowe

Overview

Definition: infection is the invasion of the body by disease causing organisms (germs). In our daily lives we pay little attention to the possibility of contracting a serious infection. There is almost an expectation that one may catch a *cold* in the winter season, and while inconvenient and uncomfortable for us, nonetheless it does not pose a serious threat to life.

Man has developed a phenomenal ability to interact with other humans, animals and the environment to enable us to enjoy a healthy existence. However this is a fine balance which, if breached, may result in disease and/or infection.

The organisms which cause disease in man are called pathogens. The essential element of this chapter is to help you safeguard your health when caring for clients with infections. This knowledge is essential for you to implement safe care for a client, without adding the risk of them acquiring a hospital-borne infection.

Key words

Micro-organism, bacteria, virus, parasite, cross-infection, commensals, disinfectants, isolation, aseptic, clean, iatrogenic, sterile, defence mechanisms, natural immunity, passive immunity, invasive procedures, pathogens, pathogenic, endogenous, exogenous.

What causes infection?

Infection is predominantly caused by small living organisms which can only be seen by the use of a microscope – hence the word *micro-organism*. Organisms can be further categorized along the lines of a family tree (Fig. 6.1).

There are numerous names given to organisms, according to their shape, size and behaviour. *Staphylococci* live on the human skin in harmony with the individual, doing no harm while they remain in that habitat. Only about 90% of organisms are potentially harmful to man.

How do individuals keep infection free?

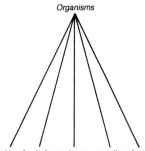

Fig. 6.1 Classification of organisms.

The *immune system* is the mechanism by which humans resist infection. Some individuals, especially those already in poor health, are considered more susceptible to infection. Humans have a complex immune system which, under most circumstances, protects against infection.

Part of the immune system is a collection of specialized cells which are transported in the blood stream and the lymphatic vessels to all parts of the body. The cells predominantly involved are the white blood cells.

The body uses physiological processes to constantly monitor for infection. If potential infection is detected the body activates the immune system to combat the invasion of pathogens. In most instances the individual will be able to recover after a short illness. However, about five hundred people in England die each year from hospital acquired infections (HAI) (Meers *et al.*, 1980).

Defence mechanisms

- Juices in our digestive tract are designed to eliminate many of the harmful organisms which we ingest. The juices alter along the digestive tract to ensure potentially harmful organisms are destroyed. For example, hydrochloric acid is produced in the stomach; most organisms are destroyed by acid.
- Tears constantly bathe the surface of our eyes to flush away organism-laden dust particles.
- Intact skin is a huge body defence against invasion by organisms. Keeping the skin in good condition and free from cuts is an important aspect of prevention of infection. Patients who develop decubitus ulcers (pressure sores) in fact have the wound infected by organisms, thus making the healing process considerably more difficult.

Immunity

Once the body has been exposed to a harmful (pathogenic) organism it usually produces an antibody cell to oppose and overcome that specific organism. If the person is exposed at a later time to the same organism, the antibody cell will *remember*, and immediately multiply to combat this invasion.

It is only pathogenic organisms which are a potential danger to man; that is to say those organisms which are capable of causing disease. The human body has many organisms which aid body functions while they are restricted in a specific area. For example, vitamin K production in the intestines is aided by bacterial activity. Such organisms are known as *commensals* or *normal flora*. Should the organisms become colonized in another area of the body they are capable of causing an infection. Colonization means the organisms multiply and flourish. For example,

Escherichia coli, a commensal organism normally found in the bowel, may cause infection if it is transmitted to the bladder or a wound.

Susceptibility of an individual to infection depends on the virulence of the organism, the number of organisms and the state of the individual's immune system.

Sources of pathogenic transmission

The source of pathogenic organisms may be:

- Humans
- Insects
- Animals
- Inanimate objects

Humans

As previously discussed, numerous organisms are commensals and may be passed to another individual by direct or indirect contact. If an individual, be they nurse or client, has an infection, they may infect another individual by cross-infection, whether in the incubation phase, acute phase or convalescent period of the infection. Some individuals are carriers of particular organisms which do not cause infection in the carrier but harm others. For example a carrier of *Staphylococcus aureus* in their nose will not show signs of infection. However, the carrier is potentially harmful if caring for new-born babies. It is sometimes necessary for staff who work with vulnerable clients to have regular nasal swab tests to check they are free from infection.

Animals

Animals may cause infection in several ways. The most common mode is when the creature is consumed. Poultry is notorious for carrying the salmonella organism, which may cause food poisoning in humans.

Insects

The mosquito bite is the cause of malaria in some parts of the world.

Inanimate objects

The soil, water and air are all capable of supporting organisms. The tetanus organism inhabits the soil. *Vibrio cholerae*, which causes cholera, inhabits some water supplies. *Legionella pneumophila*, the cause of Legionnaire's disease, can inhabit water and air cooling systems in buildings.

Modes of pathogenic transmission

There are two modes of transmission: *direct* and *indirect*.

Direct transmission

Contact between humans

This is an area where the carer needs to ensure that their own hygiene and habits are scrupulous, so as not to convey either their own organisms, or those of other clients, to another.

Inadequate hand washing between each client contact can lead to the spread of infection. For example, hands may become contaminated when emptying a urinary catheter bag, therefore it is essential to wash one's hands after each client contact. Even better, wear disposable gloves and wash your hands after any such procedure.

Inoculation transmission

This is a risk in an accidental sharps injury. It is a particular risk when the damaging object, such as a needle or scalpel blade, is contaminated with blood or body fluid. This is one way of contracting hepatitis B.

Sexual contact

This is yet another mode of direct spread. As it is not an important aspect in the nursing of clients, it will not be dealt with any further in this text.

Indirect transmission

There are numerous modes of spread and each one will be dealt with separately.

Droplet spread

This may occur when speaking, coughing or sneezing. Small water particles are formed and then sprayed into the atmosphere during these activities. These droplets as they are called may carry pathogenic or commensal organisms which another individual inhales. For example, the common cold is usually spread by droplet infection. A wound can be infected from a carer's commensal organisms which inhabit their nose and throat. It is therefore desirable to limit conversation during a wound dressing procedure.

Vectors

This term refers to a carrier such as flies and cockroaches.

Fomites

This mode of infection is via inanimate objects. These are so numerous that it is important for the carer to understand the mode of transmission, rather than the objects involved. Examples include:

- Carers' uniforms
- Bedpans
- Eating utensils

- Toiletries
- Bedclothes

and all manner of equipment that may be used in the client's care.

This is an area for significant concern as many of the procedures carried out in the work area are designed to prevent this mode of infection. For example, the wearing of a single use, disposable apron for stripping the linen off a used bed, to prevent contamination of clothing which may be in contact with a client later on.

Activity 6.1 ■

 Consider one client you have cared for and list the inanimate objects that could cause the spread of infection.

■ ■

Your list may include the following:

- Bedclothes
- Polythene washing bowl
- Bed cradle

- Pillows
- Flannel

Airborne

The air is able to suspend many organisms, thus facilitating the inhalation of organisms when we breathe. Therefore, one endeavours to reduce air currents in the work area to a minimum. It is essential to have fresh air, but not a draught. For example, fold the bed linen when stripping a used bed, as shaking and pulling create an air current and increase the circulation of organisms.

Vulnerability to infection

Some individuals are more likely than others to succumb to an infection. Many of the factors predisposing the individual to this phenomenon are well known (Fig. 6.2).

Activity 6.2 ■

 Before reading on, spend a few minutes thinking of the factors you can identify which predispose people to infection.

■ ■

Now read on and see how many you were able to identify.

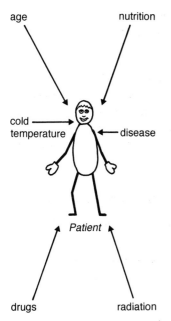

Fig. 6.2 Factors which increase the risk of infection.

Age

At either end of the continuum one is less able to resist infection. The very young have an immature immune system, while the elderly tend to have an immune system which can no longer respond rapidly to infection. For example, food poisoning may give an otherwise healthy person severe diarrhoea and vomiting, but could well prove fatal for the elderly or the young.

Nutrition

Malnutrition predisposes individuals to infection as they are unable to produce antibodies effectively. This is especially true when there is a lack of protein in the diet.

Low temperature

Exposure to temperatures which reduce the core body temperature to below normal is thought to suppress antibody production. For example, the exposure of wounds and the use of solutions reduce the healing capacity for several hours.

Disease

Individuals who are already ill may have an inefficient immune system, increasing their susceptibility to infection. This applies especially to individuals suffering from diseases such as diabetes mellitus, cancer or AIDS.

Drugs

Some drugs, especially the corticosteroids (e.g. prednisolone), while essential for some disease control, nonetheless suppress antibody production. For example, clients receiving chemotherapy drugs for the treatment of cancer are more susceptible to infection because of their drug regime.

Radiation

Exposure to therapeutic doses of radiation reduces the body's ability to produce antibodies and white blood cells.

Care of clients with infections

One aim is to increase the client's resistance to the infection. They are likely to need a nutritious diet, high in calories and protein. The client frequently does not feel like eating and drinking, so the carer needs to be

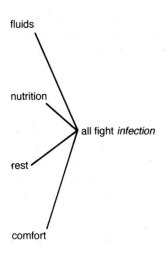

Fig. 6.3 Factors which help in the fight against infection.

imaginative in finding tempting morsels. Often special high calorie and protein drinks are ideal; perhaps these could be made into ice blocks for the patient to suck, or if the taste is unpalatable provide a drinking straw.

Because the client usually has a raised body temperature they require extra fluid to replace that lost by sweating. This is likely to be about 2500 to 3000 ml per day. The carer can, by encouragement, do a great deal to ensure the client consumes this large volume of fluid. Help the client to rest as much as possible by promoting an environment conducive to sleep. Comfort is important so change damp bed linen as necessary. Cotton night attire is best as it causes the least sweating.

The client may feel alternately hot and cold as body temperature fluctuates. A fan and/or cool washes will help in the hot flush period, and the provision of blankets when the patient feels cold. It is important to prevent shivering as this consumes a lot of energy.

Figure 6.3 illustrates a number of factors which help fight infection.

Inflammation

This is the body's response to infection and may be observed by the carer. If any of the symptoms shown in Fig. 6.4 are observed, or mentioned by the client, it is important to inform the registered practitioner. These signs and symptoms are the result of the immune response and evidence that the body is responding to the pathogens, and trying to combat the infection and destroy the harmful organisms.

Management of a client with an infection

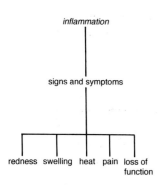

Fig. 6.4 Signs and symptoms of inflammation.

The aim of the care is not only to allow the client to recover, but also to prevent the spread of the infection to others: yourself, other staff or other clients. It is also important that the infected client is not exposed to another infection caused through inadequate preventive care. This latter type of infection is referred to as cross-infection and hospitalized patients are especially vulnerable to contracting such infections. However, with vigilance to personal hygiene and the correct carrying out of procedures, the risks can be considerably reduced.

Source isolation nursing

If the client already has an infection which is virulent, that is to say the pathogen is extremely likely to cause an infection in another, then they may be *isolated* in the hope of preventing such spread. For example, some clients who have a severe wound infection or tuberculosis will be isolated. The ward manager will ascertain who is safe to care for this client. In general, if you have been immunized for tuberculosis then you can safely care for the client.

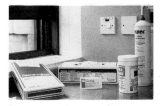

Fig. 6.5 Sample of products available for reducing the risk of contamination from harmful micro-organisms.

Specific procedures will be followed for clients in isolation regarding the disposal of waste materials and the movement of personnel and equipment out of the nursing area. Refer to the local policy for specific details to ensure safe practice.

Protective isolation

Other clients in isolation are those receiving *special drug therapy* which greatly reduces their ability to produce antibodies and other immune defence mechanisms. These clients are susceptible to contracting infection from anybody or anything with which they come into contact. They are nursed in rooms where the ventilation and temperature are ideally controlled.

All inanimate objects entering the area will be *sterile*. A sterile object is one that is free from all organisms. There are various ways to make objects sterile, usually involving heat, disinfectant or radiation treatment. Personnel will usually wear protective sterile clothing, and possibly masks, to prevent the client receiving any of their airborne or droplet organisms (Fig. 6.5).

Common risk factors for clients in hospital

- Shared facilities and equipment
- Contact with hospital staff
- Invasive procedures, e.g. surgery
- Mass-produced food
- High psychological stress factors
- Intravenous infusion

Prevention of cross-infection

- Hospital organizational policies and approaches designed to reduce infection
- Individualized client care
- Staff and client education

Individualized client care

This is achieved by assessing each individual, recording the assessment and planning the care accordingly. The care plan should always be consulted before care is given and the subsequent outcome of the care should be recorded. This enables efficient evaluation and monitoring of the client's condition.

Likewise if a system of client allocation is practised it helps to reduce the number of personnel who come into contact with the client, thus reducing the client's risk of contracting an infection.

Hospital organizational policies and procedures

These should be current and available as guides to staff practices.

Activity 6.3 ■

Identify the following in your work area: infection control policy, procedure manual.

■ ■

Staff and client education

Clients may contract an infection from either themselves, termed *endogenous*, or from other sources, termed *exogenous*.

Endogenous infections frequently arise because the client is unaware of the hazards they expose themselves to. The client's commensal organisms can be spread to cause infection. For example, *escherichia coli* from the perineum may cause a urinary tract infection in the patient who has not been taught the importance of perineal toilet following a bowel motion. The perineum is the area between the anus and the urethra (the opening to the bladder). This is especially important for the female client as their urethra is short and therefore in close proximity to the anus. It is important to teach patients to clean their perineal area from front to back, thus preventing contamination from the anus.

Clients whose hands are contaminated with organisms may peel up the corner of their wound dressing to have a look and, in the process, contaminate their wound. Teaching clients good hygiene habits and helping them to carry them out is part of the carer's role.

Activity 6.4 ■

Record the facilities available for your clients to wash their hands following toileting.

■ ■

For mobile clients these should include:

- Hot running water
- Soap individually dispensed
- Hand drying facilities with disposable towels

For bed bound clients these should include:

- Clean bowl of hot water
- Disposable flannel
- Client's own soap
- Hand towel

Exogenous infections are those acquired from others and/or the environment. *The single most important preventive measure is scru-*

Fig. 6.6 Good hand washing technique.

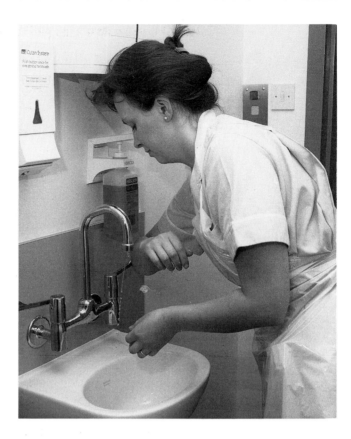

pulous hand washing and drying technique by all personnel (Fig. 6.6). Refer to your local policy for details.

General principles of hand washing

Taps can be heavily contaminated with organisms. It is important to use elbow taps correctly when they are available, i.e. turn the taps on and off using your elbows, or disposable paper towel, as this reduces the level of contamination on the taps and prevents recontamination of your freshly washed hands.

According to Ayliffe *et al.* (1982), the general technique for hand washing is:

- Remove wrist watch and jewellery
- Use hot running water to dampen your hands
- Use the correct amount of individually dispensed soap solution
- Thoroughly wash all areas of your hands, including under rings
- Rinse off soap
- Dry your hands thoroughly with disposable towels

Hand washing before and after client contact is the single most important practice in the prevention of cross-infection. Clients' personal effects should not be loaned to other patients. Facecloths and soaps should be allowed to dry between usage as this helps to reduce the environmental conditions which most organisms need for growth, i.e. dampness and darkness.

Single-use items

Single-use, disposable items should be used whenever possible. However, this may be cost prohibitive or not accepted current practice. It is the carer's responsibility to make items available for the client and to ensure they are aware of safe usage and disposal.

Activity 6.5 ■

In your work area, what facilities are available for clients to use headphone sets to listen to the radio? Are the ear pieces disposable and changed, or cleaned if not disposable, between each client?

Activity 6.6 ■

Is there an electric razor for communal use in your work area? Consider how the razor head is cleaned between each use. Identify the policy for cleaning such equipment in your work area (Millward, 1992).

■ ■

If material is not disposable but needs to be shared, then it is essential for the carer to understand the proper care for the equipment to prevent cross-infection. On the whole, the use of general purpose detergent and hot water for washing, followed by thorough drying, is appropriate for cleaning beds, bed cradles, etc., to control infection. Refer to your own organizational policy.

The environment

All carers have a responsibility to ensure that the environment within which they work is as clean as possible, to prevent the growth of organisms. Damp, dark, unclean areas support colonization; Florence Nightingale identified the importance of eradicating such conditions.

Pathogens may grow wherever there is spillage of blood, pus, urine, vomit or faeces. Therefore prompt and appropriate disposal of these is essential. In all instances the carer must ensure their hands are washed on completion of the task. Whenever dealing with a patient's body fluids it is advisable to wear disposable gloves. For information on the correct type of glove, refer to your local policy.

The carer should at all times consider their colleagues and co-workers, who may also be at risk of infection. The laundry staff are at risk from contaminated linen unless the carer has packaged the linen in the correct way.

Activity 6.7 ■

Investigate, using the policy manual as an aid, the correct packaging of the following items:

- Used linen
- Infected linen
- Linen soiled with urine, blood, etc

■ ■

Sharps

Accidental inoculation is a minor risk if policies are adhered to, but a major risk if policies are blatantly ignored.

Activity 6.8 ■

Identify your work area sharps policy and compare this with the actual practice. If there are any discrepancies discuss them with the work area manager.

■ ■

Remember that the handling of sharps in the clinical area is only the initial part of the process. The porterage and disposal will involve a considerable number of personnel who are all at risk of an accidental inoculation.

Activity 6.9 ■

Identify what to do if an inoculation injury occurs in your work area. To whom is it reported? Where is the incident recorded? What treatment is the person likely to require?

■ ■

Some employers offer their employees hepatitis B vaccination via the occupational health department. It is worth enquiring, if you are not already vaccinated.

Waste disposal

The correct disposal of waste from the clinical area is good practice, so it is essential for staff to be fully aware of the relevant policies. Again the carer is only the initial contact in the chain for disposal of waste (Fig. 6.7).

Fig. 6.7 Safe disposal of waste products.

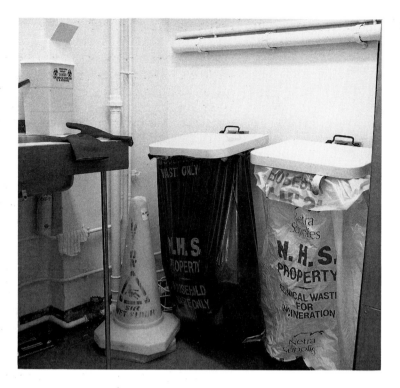

Activity 6.10 ■■■■■■■■■■■■■■■■■■■■■■■■■

 Identify the correct containers for the disposal of the following:

- Clinical waste
- Aerosols and bottles
- General waste
- Food waste

■■■■■■■■■■■■■■■■■■■■■■■■■■■■■

Spillage and cleaning

There will be domestic policies for cleaning clinical areas, which by and large will entail damp dusting so as not to create an aerosol effect. Floor cleaning will be with specially designed brooms and machines, to keep air currents to a minimum. Spillages are a hazard to staff and patients and must therefore be dealt with immediately. Small spillages can be wiped up using disposable paper towels. Larger spillages on the floor require mopping. Use clean water and an appropriate detergent to clean the area, then dispose of the water, rinse the utensils and store to enable drying.

Refer to your procedure manual for specific instructions concerning the spillage of blood.

Food handling and hygiene in clinical areas

There is a risk of clients contracting food poisoning if food is not handled safely and in accordance with the Food and Safety Act 1990. While the senior person in charge, for example the senior nurse, is responsible for ensuring safe practice is adhered to, each individual carer has a duty to care. The following principles are a guide to safe practice.

Food storage

Food may decompose or become infested or contaminated. Safe storage is therefore essential to minimize this risk in the clinical area:

- *Clean:* clinical area kitchens should be kept clean, including all storage spaces, especially the refrigerator.
- *Cool:* storage below 5°C in the refrigerator is essential. No food should be stored for more than 24 hours from when it is brought into the area, i.e. it is advisable to date food. Staff food is not to be kept in the refrigerator. No raw meat, fish, poultry or eggs should be stored in the clients' area. If food is in its original wrapper, only store until the sell by or use by date.
- *Covered:* All food must be covered and sealed, for example in a resealable plastic box. Label the box with the patient's name and the date. Once food has been served, if not consumed, it must be disposed of. Waste bins must be covered at all times with a well fitting lid.

Food handling

All personnel need to ensure their hands are washed prior to handling and serving meals. A clean disposable plastic apron is ideal to ensure one's clothing does not contaminate the food being handled. Likewise, ensure any cuts or abrasions on your hands are adequately covered. Food should be served at the correct temperature, that is 63°C or above for hot food, 5°C or below for cold food, thus reducing the risk of bacterial growth. Reheating of meals in the clients' area is to be discouraged as it is difficult to ensure that the correct temperature is achieved.

Sample collection

It may be an essential part of the carer's role to collect samples of body fluids for pathology testing to assist in establishing the client's diagnosis. All staff who come into contact with patient's body fluids should wear disposable gloves to reduce the risk of contracting an infection, in particular the HIV virus, as at the time of writing there is no known vaccine. Meanwhile, the porterage and laboratory staff may be vulnerable if the

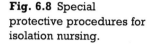

Fig. 6.8 Special
protective procedures for
isolation nursing.

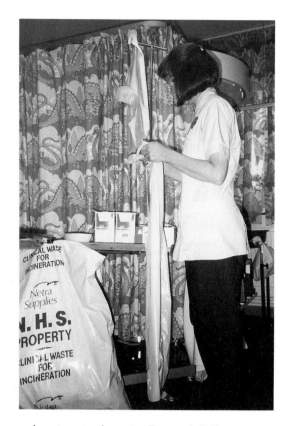

collection procedure is not adequate. Figure 6.8 illustrates some products
which help reduce the risk of contamination.

Ensure the outside of the container is not contaminated during the collection process. If contamination does occur, transfer the contents to a
fresh container. Remember, it is not adequate merely to wipe the outside of
the container clean, as the microscopic residue will remain. Ensure the lid
is securely fastened and send to pathology in accordance with your local
policy. Refer to the relevant section in Chapter 11 for more information.

Carer's health

Remember infection is a double-edged situation: you may be at risk of
contracting an infection from your work environment or, more likely, your
work practice may cause a client to succumb to an infection. The occupational health department can offer a service for monitoring the staff's
health status and providing health education. The common cold to you is a
nuisance, but to a client it could be a life-threatening chest infection.

Cuts or abrasions on your hands offer a port of entry for organisms to
establish an infection. To maintain yourself at maximum fitness it is
necessary to consume a nutritious diet and ensure adequate rest and sleep.

Summary

This chapter has provided a considerable amount of information to enable a better understanding of the modes of spread of organisms. As a carer it is essential to recognize the vulnerability of the sick and ensure safe practices to safeguard them from contracting a hospital acquired infection.

Overall, the single most important consideration in reducing the client's risk is the use of an effective hand washing technique by all carers.

References

Ayliffe, G., Collins, B. & Taylor, L. (1982) *Hospital Acquired Infection*. John Wright & Sons, London.

Food and Safety Act 1990. HMSO, London.

Meers, P., Ayliffe, G. & Emmerson, A. (1980) Report of the national survey of infection in hospitals. *Journal of Hospital Infection*, **2**, supplement.

Millward, S. (1992) The hazards of communal razors. *Nursing Times*, **88**(6), 58.

Further reading

Beaumont, G. (1992) Bad riddance to rubbish. *Nursing Times*, **88**(14), 63–4.

Bowell, B. (1992) Protecting the patient at risk. *Nursing Times*, 15 January, **88**(3), 32–5.

Curran, E. (1991) Protecting with plastic aprons. *Nursing Times*, **87**(38), 64–8.

DHSS (1987) *Health Service Catering Hygiene*. HMSO, London.

Evans, R. (1991) Child's play. *Nursing Times*, 10 June, **87**(24), 63–7.

Foodsense (1992) *The Food Safety Act 1990 and You. A Guide for the Food Industry*. Available from Foodsense, London SE99 7TT (Tel: 081-694 8862).

Gill, J. & Slater, J. (1991) Building barriers against infection. *Nursing Times*, 11 December, **87**(50), 53–4.

Greaves, A. (1985) We'll just freshen you up dear. *Nursing Times*, 6 March, **81**(10), 3–4.

Griffiths-Jones, A. (1992) The safe disposal of excreta. *Nursing Standard*, 19 February, **69**(22), 28–9.

Hart, S. (1992) Ensuring the safe disposal of sharps. *Nursing Standard*, 4 March, **6**(24), 29–30.

Linden, B. (1991) Protection in practice . . . wearing gloves. *Nursing Times*, 13 March, **87**(11).

McCulloch, J. (1992) Control of infection: points to remember. *Nursing Standard*, 25 March, **6**(27), 28–30.

McKeowan, M. (1992) Sharpening awareness. *Nursing Times*, **88**(14), 66–7.

Smith, F. (1991) Looking into the refrigerator. *Nursing Times*, **87**(38), 61–2.

Ward, K. (1992) Why not wash? *Nursing Times*, 10 June, **88**(24), 68–9.

Section 2
Endorsements for Direct/Acute Care

Chapter 7
Meeting the Elimination Needs of the Client
Christine Cooper

Overview

The chapter will consider normal elimination and the psychological, social and cultural influences on this. The use of equipment when assisting clients is outlined. How excreta are examined visually by carers to detect abnormalities and how specimens are obtained, are described. Problems with elimination, such as diarrhoea, constipation and incontinence, and how to resolve them, are considered. The chapter concludes with catheter care and some other problems with elimination in brief.

Key words

Normal elimination, privacy, specimens, abnormalities, problems, incontinence.

Normal elimination

We need fuel to provide growth and energy. After extracting the goodness from the food and drink we consume, we have to expel the remaining waste substances from our bodies.

Urine

The fluid urine is produced by the kidneys. They are vital organs and are positioned in the upper abdomen at the back (posteriorly).

Did you know?

The whole of the blood volume of an adult, 4 to 6 litres, is filtered for waste substances by the kidneys 60 times a day.

Urine drains from the kidneys via the ureters into a hollow muscular organ: the bladder. We normally store the urine there until it is an appropriate time to void it. This act is called micturition and is controlled by involuntary muscles and consciously by the brain.

The urethra is the tube that takes urine from the bladder to the outside of

Fig. 7.1 Urine is passed from the kidneys down the ureters to the bladder and is then voided via the urethra.

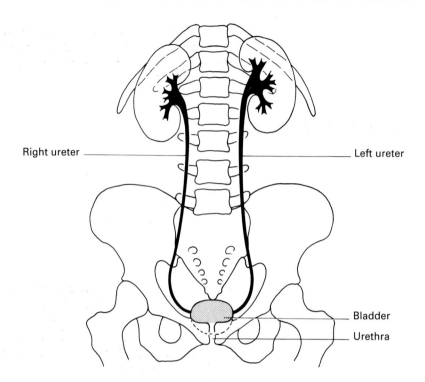

Right ureter ——— Left ureter

Bladder

Urethra

the body (Fig. 7.1). In men it is about 20 cm (8 inches) long, but in women it is only about 3.8 cm (1.5 inches). Because it is so short in women they are more likely to suffer from infections as micro-organisms have only a short distance to travel. Urine infections are commonly called cystitis. Refer to Chapter 6 on control of infection for preventive measures.

Faeces

These are formed from the waste products of food in the large bowel or colon. The large bowel is about 1.5 m (5 feet) in length. In the large bowel there are normally special bacteria which complete the breakdown process. They also help produce vitamins B and K which are necessary for the body. Water is also reabsorbed.

At the end of the colon is the rectum where faeces accumulate before being expelled out of the body through the anus. This is normally under voluntary control.

?

Did you know?

The first type of water closet (WC) was introduced in the 1500s, but failed to become established due to lack of plumbing and sewage disposal.

In 1778 Joseph Bramah patented a flush toilet, but the drainage of these in the first half of the 1800s was into cesspools which often overflowed, with unpleasant results.

Modern sewage systems were introduced in the 1860s and many of these Victorian structures are still in use today. At this time Sir Thomas Crapper made improvements to the design of WCs and they became more commonly used.

Influences on elimination

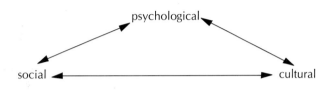

Psychological

social ← → cultural

Psychological

We learn to be independent in using the lavatory when very young. It is an important milestone in a child's life as it is often a matter of pride and praise when a child can manage for him or herself.

Therefore when clients who have been independent with regard to eliminating have to rely on carers they may suffer embarrassment and even loss of self-esteem. Imagine how you might feel having someone wiping your bottom for you. This may make them feel *like a baby*, i.e. helpless, causing feelings of distress and possible humiliation.

If this has to be done it is very important not to appear to treat the client like a child. It is essential when assisting them with elimination to preserve their *dignity* and *self-respect*.

Privacy is very important to the client who needs assistance with eliminating, as it may be stressful and embarrassing having to use strange equipment in a different environment.

Normally we eliminate in privacy behind closed doors and having to eliminate when only screened by curtains in an area like a ward, with people outside, may make clients very uncomfortable. They may be anxious about odours and might put off having to *go* because of this.

In addition, our body waste is normally flushed away without other people having to dispose of it for us, and staff removing bedpans, for example, may be another source of embarrassment. Figure 7.2 shows a toilet specially adapted to help a client be independent.

Privacy should be ensured by curtains around the client's bed area and by closing window blinds.

Try to avoid interruptions – imagine what it is like having people walking in on you when trying to *use the loo*!

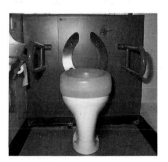

Fig. 7.2 Adapted toilet to enable a client's independence.

Cultural influences

Family behaviours are very influential on a person's habits when eliminating and these and religious beliefs must be respected.

Some cultural groups such as Muslims only use their left hand for cleaning their genitals after eliminating, keeping their right hand for eating.

If such a client is unable to use the left hand they will be unhappy about using their right and may require some assistance. Some clients may be unhappy about carers from the opposite sex assisting with such intimate care and clients' feelings should be respected. (Refer to Chapter 1 on individuality of the client.)

Social

A client's social circumstances may influence the type of facilities that they are used to. This may be important if clients are used to raised seats and hand rails or other adaptations.

Use of equipment

Activity 7.1 ■

 If you have ever been so unfortunate as to have to use a bedpan you will appreciate that they can be difficult. If not you may try just sitting on one and imagine what it is like to actually have to use one.

■ ■

Bedpans should only be used if the client cannot get out of bed to use a commode. Metal ones can be a shock to sit on if cold, so warming them first is a kindness. When taking to and from clients, a disposable paper cover should always be used over the bedpan or urinal.

Urinals may be used by male patients, but spills can occur if they are too full. Urinals should be removed for emptying after use and not allowed to become over full. Some male clients find urinating lying down very difficult and need to stand out of bed to pass urine.

After use, commodes should always be cleaned with detergent and hot water, to prevent cross-infection.

It must be remembered that the client's bed area has to function not only as a bathroom and lavatory but also a bedroom, dining room and living room.

Health and safety

Always leave clients with a call buzzer so they can summon help when needed. Clients should be sat on commodes facing the bed in case they feel faint and fall forward. Brakes must be on.

Preventing infection

After using a bedpan or commode the client should have an opportunity to wash their hands. A bowl of water should be taken to the bedside with soap and towel. The client should be repositioned and left in comfort.

Carer's personal clothing

Plastic aprons should always be worn (Fig. 7.3). Disposable gloves should be used as necessary.

Records

Complete fluid balance charts if the client's intake and output are being monitored. Also record bowel actions if required to do so. Report any abnormalities (see below).

Dealing with odours

As clients have to eliminate in areas where they often eat and spend their days, odours can be very unpleasant and embarrassing. Fresh air is best for dispelling odours, although aerosol spray is sometimes useful. However it is important to be sensitive to clients' feelings as using sprays is as good as saying 'You have caused an offensive smell'.

Checking for abnormalities

After a client has used a bedpan, commode or urinal the contents should be *checked for abnormalities* before disposal. This should be done away from the client to avoid embarrassment or causing concern.

Fig. 7.3 Protective clothing to be worn when dealing with bodily waste products.

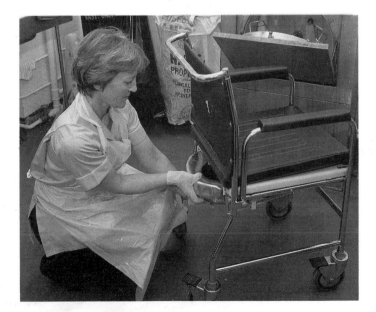

If uncertain, keep the items for inspection by a registered nurse or doctor, so cover and label with the client's name.

Any soreness or discomfort that the client experiences should be reported to the professional. The doctor may then prescribe the appropriate treatment.

Faeces

Colour
This is normally dark brown, but may be green with clear mucus in bowel disorders. There may be fresh red blood or old changed blood which makes the stool black and tarry – this may also occur if the client is taking iron tablets. Very pale or fatty looking stools may also occur in disease states.

Consistency
The stools should be soft but formed.

Odour
Stools are usually unpleasant but highly offensive stools do occur in diseases of the bowel.

Contents
Stools may contain parasites or worms; these are pale in colour and may be in segments. Children may swallow small toys which are passed in stools. Occasionally adults swallow items such as tooth caps, which could be passed in stools.

Urine

This is normally pale straw coloured.

Concentration
This will vary with how much fluid the client has been drinking. If very dark it indicates that the client is dehydrated and not drinking enough. If the client is passing a large quantity (volume) of urine it may become almost clear. Urine is more concentrated in summer when we lose more body fluid by sweating and pass less urine.

Colour
Changes can occur if there is injury causing bleeding; urine may be blood stained if the client is menstruating. Some drugs can cause the urine to become very oddly coloured, e.g. bright orange.

Clarity
If the urine becomes cloudy it is a sign of infection.

Odour

Fresh, normally concentrated urine has little odour. However if this becomes an offensive stale fish smell it indicates infection.

Urine testing

Indications for urine testing

(1) When a client is admitted to hospital. Occasionally this may indicate a disease like diabetes mellitus which the client is, as yet, not aware of.
(2) Before operations.
(3) If the client is taking certain drugs which may cause side effects; for example, bleeding may occur if anticoagulants are taken.
(4) Diabetics may test their own urine.

If you need a *specimen* of urine from a client, explain carefully what you require. Use a clean specimen jar or plastic jug that is only used for urine. If the client leaves it for you, make sure it is labelled so that there is no danger of mixing it up with other specimens.

Procedure

- Urine must be tested when it is fresh as it changes with the passage of time and this can give false results.
- Ensure that your hands are clean and dry. Disposable gloves may be worn.
- Only use reagent containers that have been kept closed. Moisture in the air causes the sticks to deteriorate. Check that the container has not passed its expiry date.
- Remove a stick carefully and replace the lid immediately. Do not touch the coloured squares of the stick with your hand or put it down on a wet surface. Often moisture from seemingly dry hands can give false results.
- The stick should be dipped in the urine, removed, then tapped lightly on the rim of the container to remove excess urine.
- You should then read the stick at the time stated in the manufacturer's instructions (Fig. 7.4).

The results: what do they mean?

pH

This is an expression of how acid or alkaline the urine is (7 is neutral, above is alkaline, below is acid). A normal reading is usually 5 to 8. Vegetarians usually have more alkaline urine, around pH 8.

Fig. 7.4 Testing urine.

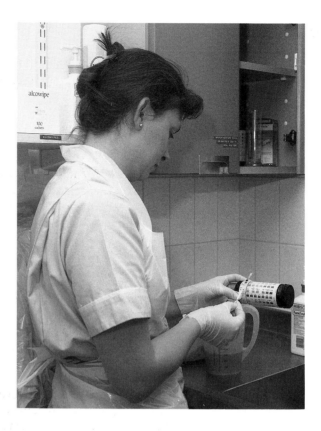

Blood
This may be seen due to trauma, menstruation in females or some drugs.

Glucose
The presence of sugar could indicate diabetes mellitus. However, further tests would be necessary before a diagnosis is made.

Ketones
These occur as the result of the breakdown of fats to produce energy when the body cannot use sugars, for example in diabetes or starvation.

Urobilinogen and bilirubin
These are abnormalities associated with liver problems.

Protein
This occurs in infections and when there has been kidney damage. It can also occur in pregnancy as a complication known as pre-eclamptic toxaemia.

Specimen collection

Specimens must always be correctly labelled and dispatched as soon as possible to the laboratory. Always wear disposable gloves.

Stool specimen

This is taken in cases of infection or to test for blood. Parasites such as worms may need identification. Occasionally specimens may be required over a number of days, sometimes all the stools passed in that time. Special large containers are then required.

Urine specimen

Midstream specimen
The first part of the stream is discarded as it may contain contaminating cells which give false results. The client must be carefully instructed, as to some it is quite a complicated procedure. First they should clean them-selves from the front to back with cotton wool and sterile normal saline. They then pass a small amount of urine, stop and then pass urine into the specimen jar. They must not contaminate the inside of the sterile specimen jar with their fingers as this will give false results.

This investigation is to determine which organism(s) is/are causing the infection so that the correct antibiotic can be given.

It may be necessary to assist clients who have difficulty in understanding the instructions. A commode without a bedpan can be used, with the carer catching the required part of the stream in a sterile jug.

Early morning specimen
This specimen is collected from the first voiding on waking. The urine is most concentrated and may be required when abnormal cells are looked for.

Twenty-four hour urine collection
The total urine passed in a 24 hour period is collected. A starting time must be identified, e.g. 6.00 AM. The first urine passed is discarded, then all urine passed during the following 24 hours is saved. Special large containers are required, sometimes with preservatives. These specimens are often required when estimating kidney function, or for sophisticated chemical or hormone tests.

A final note about specimens. Although you may become used to col-lecting excreta, clients and their visitors may not be used to seeing it. So place specimens, prior to dispatch to the laboratory, away from the public gaze and not on the tops of lockers or desks.

Constipation

This is a common problem but can often be prevented. It occurs not only in those who are unwell but also when people have a change of environment, such as admission to hospital.

Constipation may be either excessively hard stools which are difficult to pass or infrequent actions which are hard and dry. Either way, straining may result causing discomfort which is undesirable in clients who are unwell, especially those with heart problems.

Traditionally people have used laxatives to resolve the problem, often on a regular basis. However they are best avoided, unless more natural methods prove ineffective.

Activity 7.2 ■

List some foods you know that can prevent or resolve constipation.

■ ■

Your answer might include:

- Fruit such as apples, oranges and bananas
- Bran cereals
- Brown rice
- Drinking plenty of fluids (not alcohol)
- Wholemeal bread
- Vegetables

Fresh air and exercise are important too, as are having the facilities to have one's bowels open when one has the urge.

So problems are likely to occur if the client is unable to go to the lavatory when they want to. The client may eat or drink little because of feeling unwell and lack exercise because of being less mobile or confined to bed.

If laxatives or aperients are required they should normally only be a short-term measure (unless medically indicated), as excessive use will weaken the bowel muscle making constipation more likely.

The aim of using laxatives and aperients is either to soften the stool and add bulk or to stimulate the gut wall into activity. If these are ineffective other measures may be used:

- *Suppositories* – these are semi-solid or solid pellets (e.g. of glycerine) which soften the stool to make passage easier. One or two are inserted into the rectum and allowed to dissolve.
- *Enemas* – the bowel is stimulated to empty by the introduction of a volume of warm water or specially prepared fluid. An enema given to empty the bowel is called an *evacuant*.
- *Impacted faeces* – faeces which are so hard they cannot be passed are called *impacted*. An enema of oil or phosphate may be given to soften the faeces. Evacuation may then occur, or manual removal may be

performed by experienced nurses or medical staff. This must be undertaken with great care to avoid damage to tissues of the rectum.

All such treatments can be very uncomfortable and distressing. It is important not to expose the client unnecessarily and to support the client during such procedures.

Commodes and bedpans should be at hand as incontinence may occur if the client feels they must rush to go.

Diarrhoea

Most people have at some time or other experienced diarrhoea, which is at the least unpleasant. It is the passage of watery or unformed stools, often at frequent intervals and accompanied by abdominal pain and discomfort.

Activity 7.3 ■

 Identify some causes of diarrhoea which you know. Think of situations in which you may have suffered this uncomfortable problem.

■ ■

You may have included the following in your list of causes:

■ Stressful events may disturb normal bowel function and cause diarrhoea
■ Infections of the gut such as salmonella, (food poisoning)
■ Intolerance of foods and milk feeds
■ Antibiotics may cause diarrhoea as they destroy protective bowel bacteria and this allows other organisms to cause infection
■ Severe constipation with faecal impaction may result in diarrhoea leaking around the obstruction. This is called *impaction with overflow*

If diarrhoea occurs a specimen of stool will be required to check for infection. Use disposable gloves and be extra careful with handwashing. Clients with diarrhoea are often isolated in hospitals or homes to prevent spread. Diarrhoea causes fluid loss and the body becomes dehydrated. Important salts such as sodium and potassium are also lost. Particularly vulnerable to fluid loss are the very young and the elderly.

Fluids must be replaced when clients have diarrhoea and drinks should be given regularly. In extreme cases an intravenous infusion may be required. All fluids given should be measured and recorded, along with the frequency of bowel actions.

Diarrhoea is likely to be very distressing for the client, as the urge to open the bowels can be quite intense. Urgency is required to provide a commode or bedpan as quickly as possible to prevent incontinence. Much reassurance is also required to assist in alleviating distress.

Incontinence

As men draw near the common goal
Can anything be sadder,
Than master of his soul
Is servant to his bladder

Anonymous
The Speculum, Melbourne
(No. 140, 1938)

Incontinence occurs when a person has lost control of elimination and passes urine or faeces at socially inappropriate times or places.

Babies are *allowed* to soil themselves but young children are quickly encouraged to become *trained*. Incontinence then becomes a source of embarrassment and humiliation and this increases as children grow into adults. Someone with this problem is then likely to be socially isolated. There is a fear of soiling clothes in public and distressing odours.

Although the elderly and disabled are the usual age groups associated with this problem, it may occur at any age. In some cases there is little that can be done to improve or resolve the situation, such as those with severe senile dementia or those who are terminally ill.

A positive attitude is essential as much can be done, if not to resolve the problem, at least to manage it effectively so that the client is in control of the situation.

Activity 7.4 ■

Try to identify some causes of incontinence you already know about.

■ ■

Here are some examples:

- Muscular weakness of the pelvic floor which is related to childbearing in women, maybe in mothers who did not persist with postnatal exercises
- Obstruction, such as in men with enlarged prostate glands
- Nerve damage, such as spinal injury
- Client with learning difficulties (mental handicap)
- Emotional causes (fear, anxiety)
- Confusion, which may be acute or associated with senile dementia
- Institutional, where negative attitudes have induced the problem

Problems encountered – and solutions

There may be complete loss of control or just minimal soiling and/or dribbling of urine. As clients may be embarrassed and upset we may want to reassure them. However simple phrases such as 'We don't mind – we are used to it', 'Don't worry, we don't have to wash the sheets', although well meaning don't allow the client to express feelings – they do *mind* very much. So it is important to let *them say how they feel* and talk about it if they wish.

Clients should be cleaned carefully and fresh nightwear or clothes given. Some writers do not recommend the use of soap with either urinary or faecal incontinence. Water alone may be more effective. Absorbent incontinence pads and protective sheeting may be used on the bed, but care must always be taken that these do not interfere with the action of pressure sore relieving aids such as special mattresses.

Soiled personal linen must be put in plastic bags and labelled for visitors to launder at home, unless washing machines exist in the area.

Institutional linen should be placed in the appropriate soiled linen bags so that it can be dealt with correctly in the laundry.

Equipment

There is a great range of special pads and pants which can be purchased, but clients may be embarrassed to buy them. Sanitary pads may be chosen instead of using the appropriate type of appliance and padding, which often increases self-confidence. Clients need the opportunity to select and try suitable aids for themselves. You may be able to contact a continence advisor for help.

Treatment of the cause is possible and should always be considered. Surgery is one option in the case of prostate problems. Exercises can be very effective where weak muscles are the problem. Encourage clients to stop and start a few times when they pass urine as this improves muscle tone. This is something we can all do to prevent problems later in life! Have a go – it can easily become a good habit.

For clients who are confused don't wait until they become incontinent, walk or take them to the lavatory by chair at regular intervals during the day. At night walking to the lavatory might not be possible and bedpans or commodes should be offered. These measures can effectively re-establish good habits and also help prevent constipation.

Urinary catheters

These are used when clients are unable to either pass or control their flow of urine. They may be used as a temporary measure or be needed in some circumstances for long-term care.

How they work

A urinary catheter is a tube, usually about the diameter of a pen, which has a small inflatable balloon at the tip just below the eyelet for the drainage of

Fig. 7.5 The bladder showing self-retaining catheter in position (*Courtesy Bard Ltd*).

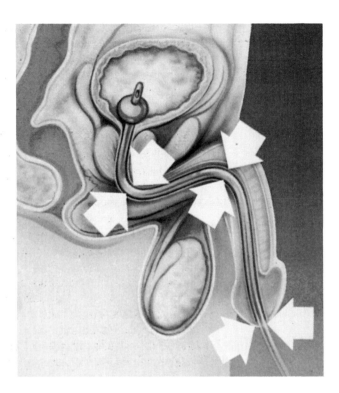

urine. This tube is passed into the bladder using aseptic technique by either a doctor or registered practitioner. The balloon is inflated with sterile water (through a small inner tube), to prevent the tube falling out (Fig. 7.5). The catheter is connected to a drainage tube and bag, creating a closed system for collecting urine and preventing organisms entering the bladder.

This seems such a simple and effective way of solving the problem, why is it not used for all clients who are incontinent? Well, catheters are not without problems: they can cause serious infections, damage to the urethra and can be uncomfortable. Having your urine draining into a bag for everyone to see is not exactly good for self-esteem!

The decision to catheterize is not taken without careful assessment of the situation. It would be preferable to try all other means to investigate and treat urinary incontinence before resorting to a catheter. However where this solution becomes inevitable, for example in a client with multiple sclerosis or spinal injury, immaculate care must be given to reduce risks to the minimum.

Keeping catheters clean

The area around the catheter where it enters the body must be kept clean to avoid infection. When cleaning, wipe away from the body down the tube. The care plan will provide instructions with regard to cleaning materials, either sterile normal saline and sterile gauze swabs or unperfumed soap and water.

Observe for discharge around the catheter. Also check for leakage which sometimes occurs if the catheter is the wrong size. Any discharge or leakage must be reported.

Keeping the catheter secure

Any pulling on the catheter will cause pain and discomfort. This can be avoided if the catheter is carefully taped to the client's leg, but it should not be too tight. Never pin the catheter to the bed clothes as this restricts movement and may cause trauma.

The tubing must not become twisted or kinked or it will fail to drain. If the bag is lifted urine must not flow back up into the bladder; pinching the tubing with the fingers or clamping when the bag has to be lifted can prevent this.

The drainage bag should not drag on the floor as this will increase the likelihood of infection. It should be attached to the bed, a stand or the client's leg if a leg bag is used.

The bag should be emptied at regular intervals, usually at least three times a day or to fit with the client's personal routine (Fig. 7.6). The carer should wear disposable gloves for this procedure and the urine is carefully

Fig. 7.6 Emptying urine drainage bag.

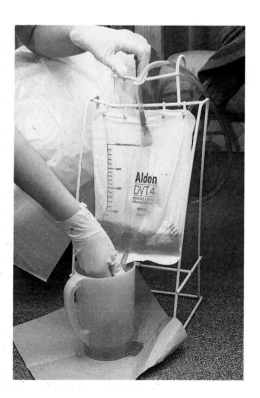

emptied into an appropriate container such as a plastic jug used only for this purpose. Care must be taken when opening and closing the drainage valve not to contaminate it.

Bags should be changed daily or as required and great care must be taken to avoid contamination when disconnecting the catheter to connect it to a new bag. For mobile patients leg bags can be used which provide a more discrete and less restricting option (Fig. 7.7).

Some special terms connected with elimination

Stress incontinence

This is a problem of urinary incontinence related to muscle weakness. If the client laughs, coughs or sneezes pressure is exerted on the bladder and urine is forced downwards, weak muscles relax and urine is voided. This can cause great embarrassment and make the client fear social outings. Imagine the humiliation of wetting yourself in public!

Muscle tone can sometimes be improved by electrical stimulation treatment given by the physiotherapist, but best results are usually obtained from corrective surgery.

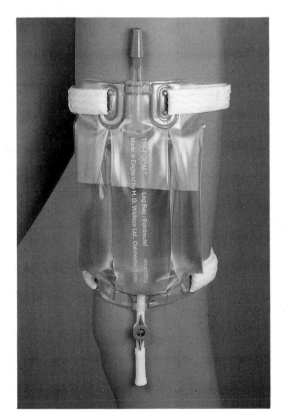

Fig. 7.7 Disposable leg drainage bag (*Courtesy Smith Industries Medical Systems*).

Colostomy

Colostomy or stoma is the raising of a loop of large bowel (colon) to the surface of the abdominal wall. Faeces can then pass out of this opening into a disposable plastic bag or dressing applied to the stoma.

The stoma is created surgically to relieve obstruction due to disease or cancer. The colostomy may be temporary or permanent. Whichever applies, special care and management are required.

Ileostomy

This is similar to colostomy but the stoma (opening) is into the small bowel. The faecal discharge is therefore fluid and contains enzymes which are destructive to skin. Therefore careful application of disposal bags and meticulous skin care are essential.

Haemorrhoids (piles)

These are grossly enlarged (varicose) veins of the anal canal. They may be inside or outside. They are caused by straining due to constipation or by raised intra-abdominal pressure, due for example to excess weight or pregnancy.

Treatment may be with special creams, relief of constipation, weight reduction, birth of baby or, in severe cases, surgery.

Summary

Removal of body waste is an essential function. For those who are unable to meet their own elimination needs unaided, it is important that carers maintain dignity and promote self-esteem for clients, giving skilled and sensitive care.

References

Gooch, J. (1989) Skin hygiene. *Professional Nurse*, **5**(1), 13–18.

Further reading

Gould, D. (1985) Management of indwelling urethral catheters. *Nursing Mirror*, **161**(10), 17, 18, 20.
King, M. (1984) Aids for incontinence, *Nursing Mirror*, **158**, 30–1.
Moody, M. (1990) *Incontinence, Patient Problems and Nursing Care*. Heinemann, Oxford.

Norton, C. (1986) *Nursing for Continence*, Beaconsfield Publications, Beaconsfield.

Roper, N. Logan, W. & Turney, A. (1990) *The Elements of Nursing*, 3rd edn. Churchill Livingstone, Edinburgh.

Chapter 8
Hygiene and the Client
Christine Cooper

Overview

This chapter explores attitudes to hygiene considering cultural, economic, family and peer group influences. Patient choice and personal rights along with nakedness and privacy and the attitudes of both the carer and the client are all discussed. The feeling of dependency and the experience of being unable to look after oneself are also considered.

The chapter discusses body image and clients' responses and how care should be given according to a care plan. It also covers the location of where hygiene needs should be met, from bed areas to the bathroom, considering in this respect health and safety aspects, infection control and the dependency of the client.

Key words

Hygiene, privacy, dependency, social interaction, body image, mouth care, cosmetics, infestation.

Attitudes to personal hygiene

Daily washing and bathing routines are very personal but will also be influenced by a number of factors (see Fig. 8.1).

Activity 8.1 ■

 Using Fig. 8.1 as a guide, make a list of factors that influence your personal hygiene routines.

■ ■

Your list may contain some of the following:

Family influences

We start our lives by being washed by our guardians, usually mothers, and many people carry on routines learned in childhood. Family habits vary;

Fig. 8.1 Factors influencing attitudes to personal hygiene.

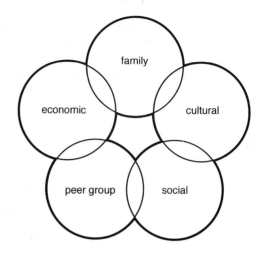

some bath daily, others bath weekly. How many of us were made to clean our teeth morning and night by caring mothers, though we may not have thought they were so caring at the time.

Economic

Individuals may ask 'Can I afford to heat the water, the cost of soap . . .?' How well off you are may well be reflected in your washing facilities.

Peer groups

Many people, especially the younger generation, are strongly influenced by group pressures and attitudes to personal hygiene and are moulded by friends and those whose opinions they value.

Social isolation

Those who have very little contact with others, either by choice or personal circumstances, for example the elderly, disabled and housebound people and those who receive few visitors, may be less motivated to pay attention to *personal hygiene*.

Have you ever been sick on your own and not felt like bothering to wash as usual? It must be easy to think 'I never go out and meet people, so why bother to wash'.

Cultural differences

Attitudes to washing vary greatly between cultural and religious groups. Some may have strict practices and taboos. In many western countries strong body odour is considered offensive (the great selection of deo-dorants available confirms this), while in other countries body odour is normal and quite socially acceptable. In some religions a high value is placed on personal cleanliness.

It is therefore important to respect clients' *cultural attitudes* towards personal hygiene and their rights to choose and to continue their normal personal hygiene routines.

Clients' choice

When it comes to changing poor hygiene practices a balance should be struck. It is important to encourage or adapt personal hygiene routines in order to improve health and prevent infection. It also has to be remembered that in institutions where clients have to live in close contact and share communal facilities, poor hygiene practices may cause others offence or harm. In either situation carers should tactfully persuade clients to keep clean.

How often clients need to wash is a balance between their condition and the desire to promote health through cleanliness, and the need to respect their right to make an informed choice for their own personal hygiene routines.

Nakedness and privacy

Today some people expose more of their bodies than did previous generations. Many of today's elderly people rarely undressed in front of others, even their spouses. Personal hygiene was achieved by removing items of clothing and washing parts of the body one at a time. They may have washed in a tin bath in front of the fire, as many working people had no bathrooms. Bath night had to be a well organized family ritual.

Modesty is valued by some religious and cultural groups, especially women, for example Muslims.

In many institutions the bathrooms are communal; some may even have more than one bath in a room. It is essential to maintain clients' *self-respect* and ensure *privacy* when washing or bathing. Some, for example men who have experienced life in the armed services, often seem less concerned about openly sharing washrooms. But we must always be careful that we do not generalize, put people into categories and treat them the same. Privacy should always be available and respected for all those who wish it.

Protect the client's privacy

- Bed areas must always be fully screened with no gaps between curtains
- Staff should respect privacy and avoid intruding by unnecessarily opening curtains, when clients may be exposed
- Window blinds should be drawn as clients may be overlooked

Feeling dependent

Young children and babies need help from parents to wash and part of growing up is learning to care for your own body. As adults able to wash ourselves, perhaps this is something we think little about.

Activity 8.2 ■

 What is it like to be washed? With a friend or partner wash each other's hands and faces. How did it feel? Was the water too hold or cold? Was your partner gentle? Be truthful and share with each other what it was like.

■ ■

You may have felt a bit like a baby. Some clients feel very distressed at returning to a childlike state, especially if it is unlikely that they will recover full independence again. It is important to use a sensible approach, but the carer should not assume the role of a mother-like figure as this may discourage clients from regaining their independence.

A time to talk: social interaction

When assisting clients with their hygiene needs an opportunity is created to talk to the carer privately. Clients who are worried or anxious may feel more comfortable about asking difficult questions or disclosing concerns and sharing information with the carer. It is important to allow the client time and opportunity to express themselves; carers should be supportive and prepared to listen and comfort.

Carers should report back to or refer to the professional responsible for the care as appropriate, always respecting the client's confidentiality.

Body image

The term *body image* is, as it suggests, that mental picture we have of ourselves.

Activity 8.3 ■

 Consider whether you think of yourself as under- or overweight. Do you perceive yourself as others do? Try to describe your main characteristics. Are you conscious of a particular feature, such as what you consider a large nose? Have you ever looked at a photograph of yourself and said 'Is that me, do I really look like that?'

■ ■

So why do we not recognize ourselves? Is it that what we think we look like, is not quite the same as reality? An example might be the mental health disorder anorexia nervosa (which affects the person's eating habits), where the sufferer has a seriously distorted idea of themselves. They think they look fat when in fact they are very thin.

It can be distressing for clients to see an actual body change which alters the image they normally have of themselves.

Activity 8.4 ■

 Try to think of conditions or situations which may affect a client's body image.

■ ■

You may have thought of:

- Scarring
- Loss of a limb (amputation)
- Removal of a breast (mastectomy)
- Skin disorders
- Weight loss
- Hair loss
- Opening of the bowel on to the abdomen (colostomy)
- Paralysis of a limb (hemiplegia) caused by a stroke
- Damage due to wounds or burns

When assisting with hygiene needs, carers need to be aware that a client may become distressed by the sight of their altered body. The client may be embarrassed and expect negative responses on the part of the carer. It is especially important not to give this impression by non-verbal cues. The carer should be supportive, allowing the client to express their feelings as this will assist eventual acceptance of a changed body image.

How hygiene care should be given – the care plan

If the client has a perceived problem meeting hygiene needs, this will be included in the client's care plan devised by the professional. Clients may be totally dependent or only require minimal assistance. How much help is required may alter as the client's condition changes.

The care plan should indicate the following:

- What level of independence is realistically to be aimed for within a given period of time, so you will be working towards achievable goals. Some clients may always be in need of some help while others will quickly regain their former level of independence.

■ Which areas are to be cleansed and how; for example specific prescribed lotions may need to be applied.

■ If appropriate, which areas should not be washed or treated, for
example skin markings where a client is receiving radiotherapy.

Where hygiene needs are met

If clients are confined to bed, either at home or in an institution, that area
becomes not only their bedroom, but dining room, living room, bathroom
and lavatory. It is preferable to try and reduce this multi-purpose use of an
area where possible, and if the client's condition permits, use of the
bathroom should be encouraged. Movement and exercise are stimulating
as is a change of scenery, and a walk to the bathroom may afford time for
conversation with others.

Some clients who can get out of bed and have limited mobility prefer to
wash by their beds and some may require assistance in some inaccessible
areas such as their backs or feet.

Finally, clients who are too unwell to get out of bed require a bed or
blanket bath (the latter so called because a blanket is used to cover the
patient whilst they are undressed and being bathed).

Some clients may be confined to bed for a short period of time but are
able to wash in bed with minimal assistance as their mobility is not so
restricted and they have full use of their hands.

Skin care

The skin is a protective barrier that needs to be maintained intact. An
uncleaned wound, no matter how small, could lead to a debilitating
infection. The skin is the largest organ in the body and it:

■ Has a surface area of
approximately 2 square
metres (21.5 square feet)
■ Regulates body temperature
■ Excretes water and salt
■ Manufactures vitamin D

■ Receives stimuli perceived as
pain, pressure and temperature
■ Screens harmful UV rays from
the sun
■ Covers and protects inner
organs

The skin is composed of two layers: an outer epidermis of dead and
dying cells and the inner dermis (true skin) which is a strong, flexible
meshwork of fibres and structures. Figure 8.2 illustrates the many com-
ponents in an ideal arrangement.

Fig. 8.2 Section through skin.

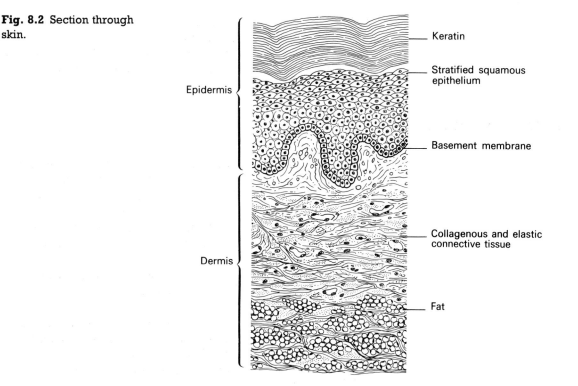

Epidermis

Dermis

Keratin

Stratified squamous epithelium

Basement membrane

Collagenous and elastic connective tissue

Fat

Dry and sensitive skin problems

Any situations or agents which reduce the water or natural oils in the skin can produce dryness and sensitivity. The following examples should be considered in particular when providing hygiene care for clients:

- *Soap and detergents* – prolonged or excessive use removes oils and causes dryness, soreness and chapping.
- *Perfumes* – can act as irritants causing dermatitis (Gooch, 1989), which results in intense itching with blisters and cracks.
- *Age* – skin becomes thinner and less elastic with age, water and sebum are reduced, skin becomes dry and wrinkled and hair and finger nails become brittle.
- *Fluid* – a reduction in body fluid may be due to drinking less or to loss from trauma or other illness.

Skin should not be rendered too dry by excessive application of drying or irritating agents. Skin moisture may be preserved by the judicious use of soap and water and by the application of moisturizing creams and oils.

Activity 8.5 ■

When washing a client you may observe skin abnormalities that require you to inform the registered practitioner. From your experience, make a list of abnormalities which you know about.

■ ■

Your list may include:

- Rashes – these may be caused by medications or contact with irritating substances; it may indicate that the client is suffering from an illness such as measles;
- Inflammation or redness – this may be a sign that a pressure sore or other infection is developing;
- Swelling or oedema – this may be due to trauma or fluid retention in the tissues caused by heart or kidney failure;
- Spots or boils;
- Dry, flaking skin;
- Bruising, cuts, burns, blisters, pressure sores;
- Insect bites.

Bathing a client

Activity 8.6 ■

Should you be dependent on someone else to meet your hygiene needs, list the points you would like them to consider when helping you.

■ ■

Your list may contain some of the following:

- Privacy
- Dignity
- Consideration of any cultural customs
- Warmth
- Gentle handling
- Skill in carrying out a procedure; keeping to a routine if at all possible
- Explanation of the procedure and the development of a relaxed atmosphere and rapport
- Education and health promotion

Preparation

- Prior to washing or bathing, the client should be offered a bedpan, urinal, commode or use of the toilet, after which handwashing facilities must be made available.

- Pain must be relieved before commencing washing or bathing. Drugs should be given by a registered practitioner and time allowed for them to take effect. This will enable the client to move or be moved without pain and bathing will be a comfortable experience.
- Unwanted items and furniture should be moved out of the way to provide a clear workspace. A chair should be available in the bathroom for the client who is unable to stand for any length of time.
- Privacy should be ensured whenever the client is washed. An engaged sign should be used on the bathroom door to prevent any unnecessary intrusion.
- When the client is washed in bed the bed height must be raised to a comfortable and safe level for the carers.
- With the client's permission collect from their locker the items required, such as soap, flannels, towels, toothpaste and brush, comb, toiletries, clean clothing and bed linen. These should be kept for that individual client's use only or disposed of. Naturally if the client has their own toiletries and washing equipment, then these should be used.

Bathing in bed

- The top bedclothes should be stripped, as the bed will need remaking and the linen may become damp.
- The top sheet is pulled down under the blanket, which is left in place to cover the client. The night clothes are then removed.
- The client is washed systematically starting, as a rule, from the face. The order for washing a client may be dependent on their specific needs. For instance, should the client have been incontinent, then the genital area will be washed first and the water and bed changed before the face is washed.
- The skin should be washed using firm but gentle strokes. After soaping, the skin is rinsed and quickly dried to prevent chilling. When drying check with the client that they feel dry.
- The water should be changed when it gets very soapy or cool.
- Check if the client normally has soap on their face before cleansing. If the client is able, he or she may wish to wash their own face. Eyes should be wiped with clean water.

Bathing specific areas of the body in bed

For *arms and hands*, start with the arm further from you, place a towel under the arm, then wash and rinse that arm and hand, paying special attention to the axilla (underarm), then wash the nearest arm. Hands may be soaked in the bowl of water, which facilitates nail care and can also be relaxing for the client. If there is an assistant with you, they can dry the arms and hands whilst you prepare to wash the next area.

The *chest and upper abdomen*: in women the area under the breasts, especially if the client is large, should be carefully washed and dried, as it can easily become sore and excoriated. Talcum powder should be applied sparingly, as it can become congealed and cause further soreness.

The *upper back* can be washed with the client sitting forward with a second person giving support if necessary. Alternatively the client can lie on their side, the towel being placed on the sheet to prevent it becoming damp, and the upper back washed.

Whilst lying on their side, the client's *buttocks* and *perineal area* (the area between the legs) can also be washed, using a specially designated flannel. Disposable flannels are preferable for this purpose. Following this the water must be changed.

The *legs and feet* are washed using the same principle as for the arms, allowing the feet to be soaked in a bowl of water if possible. Each leg should be lifted gently, supported in a cupped hand and the calves checked for pain, redness or swelling as this may indicate a deep vein thrombosis. This is a serious complication of bed rest due to immobility for a period of time.

The client should also exercise their legs and ankles. If the client is unable to move their own feet then the carer should carry out passive exercises for them.

Toilet of genital areas, if possible, should be carried out by the client for themselves. This helps to maintain dignity and independence. A second towel is placed between the legs to prevent the sheet from becoming damp and an appropriate flannel or disposable wipe is used. The carer should prepare and hand the flannel and towels to the client.

It may be necessary for you to wash the client. When assisting a female client remember to wash from front to back to avoid bacteria from the anal area contaminating the urethra and causing urinary infection. When assisting an uncircumcised male client, care should be taken to gently fold back the foreskin and wash and dry the penis before replacing the foreskin. The scrotum is also washed with care. For washing clients who are incontinent, refer to Chapter 7 to the section concerning incontinence.

When attending to a client's hygiene needs carers should observe pressure areas for any signs of the effects of excess pressure. Redness, heat or discomfort must be reported immediately to prevent skin breakdown.

After the bed bath is completed

When the client has been washed and dried they can be dressed in appropriate clothing. Take care to help them, in order to prevent the pulling of clothes over bony prominences causing friction damage to the skin.

Any soiled personal clothing should be placed in a labelled plastic bag and made available for relatives to take home to launder, or appropriate procedures followed for laundering a client's own soiled clothing.

Assisted washes

Many clients are able to undertake their own hygiene with assistance from a carer. This could be in bed, at the bedside or in the bathroom. The assistance required should have been documented in the client's care plan by the professional. It may be possible to leave the client and return to help as required. Equipment and clothing should be within easy reach and a call buzzer should be available. *Privacy*, *safety* and *warmth* should be ensured.

Baths

Activity 8.7 ■

Bathing is a common activity. Can you think of any reasons for bathing other than cleansing?

■ ■

You may have thought of:

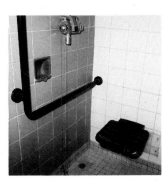

Fig. 8.3 Shower adapted to maintain independence.

- Relaxation, especially with perfumed foam or oils
- Healing, by increasing circulation to wound areas
- Refreshment: after a hard day's work
- Psychological effects of warmth and well-being

Clients should ideally be given the choice of a bath or shower and effort made to maintain their normal routine, if the client's physical condition allows and appropriate facilities are available.

Showers are very much a personal preference and some elderly people would prefer a strip wash or a soak in the bath. Showers are refreshing after sporting activities or a visit to the gym for physiotherapy. Shower chairs can be used for those unable to stand unaided. Figure 8.3 illustrates a shower adapted to maintain a client's independence.

Assisting in the bathroom

Helping the client to bath in the bathroom has been mentioned in the section on assisted washes. Note the following points:

- Consideration should be paid to general health and safety by providing a non-slip surface or rubber mat in the bath.
- A bathmat should be available for the client when they step out of the bath, either an individual or a disposable one.
- Bath water should be run prior to the client going to the bathroom and great care taken to ensure it is the correct temperature by running cold water first and adding hot water until the required temperature is reached. Scalds can easily occur, especially in the elderly who do not register hot or cold so efficiently as they get older.

The assistance a client may need will vary. The plan of care will indicate how much assistance or what handling aids are required for each client.

Fig. 8.4 Bathroom adapted to enable client's independence.

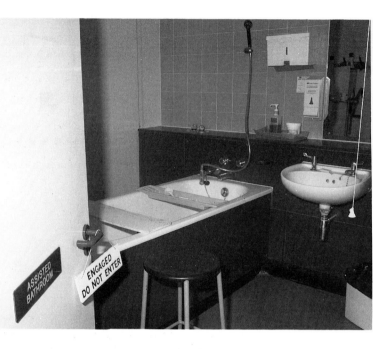

Bath seats and handles, transfer boards, stools and hoists should all be available for clients who need them (refer to Chapter 5 on mobility and safer client handling). Figure 8.4 illustrates a bathroom modified to help a client maintain independence. If the client has been incontinent it is preferable that the genital area is washed prior to their getting into the bath.

Following the bath the client is wrapped in a dry warm towel to prevent chilling and to maintain modesty. A stool should be available for them to sit on. They are carefully dried and dressed. Assistance to clean teeth and comb hair should be provided.

The client is then helped back to the ward or the day room. You should then return to the bathroom to clean the bath and remove used towels.

Mouth care

Keep your mouth wet and your feet dry

Benjamin Franklin, 1733, *Poor Richard's Almanac*

If the mouth and teeth are dry, dirty and diseased, eating and drinking become difficult and uncomfortable. Therefore the mouth should be kept moist, teeth clean and gums healthy. A dry mouth is more susceptible to infection and for clients who have diminished resistance to infection mouth care will be necessary.

?

Did you know?

The salivary glands produce about 1000 ml of saliva a day. Saliva is mostly water with a substance called lysozyme which helps to destroy bacteria. Salivary production increases at the sight and smell of food. I am sure your mouth has watered at the sight or smell of your favourite dish! Another function of saliva is that it helps break down food, thus aiding digestion. As it keeps the mouth moist it helps when chewing food (mastication) and aids swallowing. Some drugs reduce the production and flow of saliva, making the mouth unpleasantly dry, affecting eating and sometimes making talking difficult.

If the client is unable to eat or drink, mouth washes should be readily available to help keep the mouth moist (Fig. 8.5).

Care of teeth

When foods containing sugars and starches are eaten some dissolve in the saliva and are consumed by the bacteria in our mouths. This sticky mass of micro-organisms coats the teeth and is called plaque (Kahn, 1986). The bacteria produce acids which, if not removed by brushing, attack the enamel of the teeth causing holes or dental caries. Gums that support the teeth can also be affected by inflammation (gingivitis).

Losing teeth is often considered a natural part of ageing, but looking after your teeth can mean you can keep these precious items well into old age.

Equipment for cleaning teeth/mouth care

Items may include:

- Toothbrush
- Toothpaste

Fig. 8.5 Having a mouthwash.

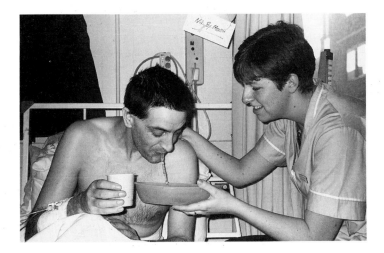

- Mouthwash
- Small gauze swabs

- Dental floss
- White paraffin or lip salve
- Cleaning lotions

Equipment should be selected according to the client's age, ability and need.

The client who is infirm and unable to clean their mouth may require special mouth care which will be identified on the care plan. Carers should watch mouth care performed by an experienced professional before undertaking the procedure.

If the client is unconscious they should lie on their side so that fluids can drain out of the mouth and breathing is not endangered. The lower side of the mouth should be cleaned, the client turned over and the other side treated. Oral suction may also be necessary to prevent excess fluid collecting in the client's mouth.

Solutions used for mouth care include:

- Sodium bicarbonate solution, to remove coating and dried mucus;
- Glycerine of thymol mouthwash, to rinse and freshen;
- A range of proprietary mouth washes;
- Paraffin or lip salve for dry lips.

Clients should be encouraged to clean their teeth morning and evening. Cleaning the mouth/teeth last thing at night is most important, as it is during the night that bacterial action and build up of plaque occurs.

Activity 8.8 ■

 Try cleaning a colleague's teeth and then ask them to clean yours. Compare notes.

■ ■

- Did you know what was happening?
- Was communication clear?
- Was it comfortable?

- Did your teeth feel clean afterwards?
- What have you learned from this experience?

Preventing a dry mouth

In illness the client may become dehydrated, especially if they have a fever. The mouth will become dry, the tongue furred, lips cracked and the risk of infection is increased. This discomfort can be prevented by careful and regular mouth care plus an adequate fluid intake as indicated in the plan of care. Fluid intake can be monitored by recording how much the client drinks on a fluid balance chart. Citrus fruit juices stimulate the flow of saliva and are refreshing, especially with the addition of ice in hot weather. Sucking ice cubes is another way of keeping the mouth moist.

Dentures

False teeth and those who wear them are often the butt of jokes. Clients, especially younger people, may be embarrassed about them.

If dentures are lost life becomes difficult; the client cannot eat solid foods and may have difficulty in speaking clearly. Also replacement is expensive. When not being worn it is important to store dentures in a labelled denture pot kept in the vicinity of the owner. Some clients prefer to remove dentures at night. Dentures should be cleaned in the bathroom using a toothbrush and under running water.

While dentures are removed the mouth can be rinsed out with a mouth wash and the gums gently massaged with a small soft toothbrush to remove any debris and to help them keep healthy; the dentures can then be replaced.

Hair care

Hair should be brushed or combed and arranged in the client's own preferred style. This should be done with care as some hair types cannot tolerate vigorous brushing. For example, for some people of African origin if their hair is not combed carefully it could tear. Some hair types may require special treatments with oil or lotions to keep them in good condition.

?

Did you know?

There are approximately 100 000 hairs on the scalp and we lose about 70–100 of these each day. A hair grows about 1 mm in three days. On the scalp this continues for about two to six years then stops and the hair falls out; a new one then starts to grow.

Illness and certain treatments such as radiation or chemotherapy (used for clients with cancer) may both increase hair loss and affect the rate of its growth.

Hair washing

Activity 8.9 ■

 How do you feel when your hair feels dirty and greasy? What would you seek to do about it and why?

■ ■

You may have identified that such a situation may have a negative effect on morale. One just does not feel good. Mood reflects on hair and hair condition reflects on mood, i.e. you feel dull and lifeless like your hair.

Self-esteem is affected by our appearance and if we already feel we cannot be bothered with our appearance, then dirty hair will have a further negative effect.

Giving the client the opportunity to wash their hair, or washing their hair for them, can be a great morale booster. I am sure you too have felt *good* with your hair clean and shiny. A client's hair can be washed in the bathroom, at the bedside or, for those confined to bed, hair can be washed in bed.

Washing hair in bed

- Remove the head of the bed and lie the client flat with their neck and shoulders well supported on pillows.
- Protect the bedclothes by placing a plastic sheet under the client's head. This will allow dirty water to drain downwards into a bucket placed at the back of the bed.
- Hairwashing trays, similar to the backwash in the hairdressers, can be used if available.
- Check the temperature of the water to be used on the inner aspect of your own wrist.
- Using a jug, gently pour a little water over the client's head and check that it is comfortable for them.
- Wet the hair thoroughly before applying shampoo, then gently massage using equal pressure from both hands, to prevent shaking the head.
- Take care to protect eyes from shampoo and water and observe the client carefully during the entire procedure.
- Rinse the hair with clean warm water and then towel dry.
- Remove water and plastic sheet.
- Replace the head of the bed then, if possible, sit the client up and dry their hair with an electric hairdryer.

If the client is able, encourage them to dry and brush their own hair in their desired style. Professional hairdressers sometimes visit clients in hospital, residential homes or in their own homes. Having hair cut, washed and styled has a greatly beneficial effect on self-esteem and morale; in fact it can, at times, provide a real boost.

Eye care

Eyes are so precious they should always be treated with care and respect. Any abnormalities observed by carers or described by the client must be reported to the registered practitioner. If a client has a discharging eye this may be an indication of infection. Following assessment, care may include taking a swab of the discharge in order to identify the causative organism. This procedure will be carried out by a registered practitioner. You may, however, be asked to carry out eye toilet to keep eyes clean.

Performing eye toilet

Hands should be washed and dried. The procedure is a clean technique. Packed sterile swabs and normal saline solution are used. Many units provide ready packed trays for eye toilet.

- The procedure is explained to the client and their consent obtained.
- The eye and the skin areas round it should be inspected and any features noted, e.g. swelling, redness.
- Using a swab soaked in normal saline, clean the eye by gently wiping from the inner aspect (by the nose) to the outer.
- Use the swab once only and discard it.
- Repeat the process until all the discharge is removed.
- Take care not to contaminate the saline solution by only placing clean swabs in it.
- Finally, use a dry swab to dry the eye and leave it comfortable.
- Dispose of the swabs and container.
- Wash and dry your hands.

Ear care

The outer ear should be cleaned with the client's own face flannel or cotton wool swabs or *buds*. If there is an excessive build-up of wax (which often occurs in the elderly client and can affect hearing) the ear(s) may need to be syringed by a doctor or registered nurse.

If a client is having problems with hearing, first look into the outer ear for signs of excess wax and, if this is observed, report back to the registered nurse so that appropriate action can be taken.

If the client has a hearing aid this should be cleaned in accordance with the manufacturer's instructions. Clients should be encouraged to wear their hearing aids, as if they cannot hear their safety is at risk. Advice concerning battery replacement and servicing of hearing aids can be obtained from audiology departments.

Nail care

Nails are hardened skin cells which protect fingers and toes. Finger nails grow at a rate of 1 mm a week, toe nails grow more slowly.

Nails should be trimmed when necessary: finger nails cut slightly rounded, toe nails cut straight across to prevent them from *in growing*. Nail clippers should be used for toe nails as these nails are harder and more difficult to cut, especially in the elderly. Soaking feet in warm water prior to cutting makes the task easier, but any client who has very hard or over-grown toe nails should be seen by a podiatrist. Clients who are diabetic should *always* be treated by the podiatrist as the risk of infection due to skin abrasion is high.

If nails are dirty, cleaning with the client's own nail brush will be necessary. Hard skin on hands and feet may be treated with oils or creams.

Activity 8.10   ■

If you are unused to cutting another person's nails, practise on a member of your family, a friend or colleague. Ask them how they found it. Practice will teach you how to hold the client's hand or foot and the angle from which to cut the nail.

■ ■

Shaving

Men for their sins have shaving too entailed upon their chins, a daily plague.

Byron, *Don Juan, Cante* XVI 23

Despite the recent fashion for designer stubble made famous by some pop stars, male clients who are not shaved daily appear unkempt. This can be distressing for the client and their visitors as it gives an *uncared for* impression. Morale and self-esteem can be greatly improved by shaving.

Male carers can draw on their own experience when shaving, but female carers may find it beneficial to practise on a willing family member or friend, who can provide feedback on how effective the shaving technique is!

Electric razors are usually quicker, but only the client's own razor should be used. The use of communal electric razors is not acceptable because of the hazard of cross-infection, in particular with blood-borne organisms.

For wet shaving, safety razors only should be used. Blades should be sharp otherwise shaving is very painful and skin may be damaged. Used blades and disposable razors should be placed in the sharps container for disposal.

Excessive hair growth should be trimmed first using clippers or scissors, as attempting to shave long facial hair is extremely painful. If the client is confined to bed they will need to be supported in an upright position with a bed table, bowl of hot water, razor, shaving soap or foam, brush, towel and mirror to hand.

Usually the client will prefer to shave himself, but if you have to do this for him then follow this procedure:

- Moisten the area to be shaved with hot water to soften the hair and skin, then apply the soap or foam.
- Gently pull the skin taut and shave using downward strokes.
- Avoid pressing too hard as this can cut the skin.
- Ask the client to move his mouth in different directions to help make the skin surface taut.
- On completion, wash off any residual soap or foam and dry the client's face.
- Cold water or aftershave may be applied at the client's request.
- Offer the mirror for him to inspect the end result.

The client with a beard or moustache may need to have these trimmed; however, permission should be obtained and it may be better to ask the assistance of a barber to do this.

Unwanted facial hair in females can be most effectively removed using depilatory creams. If the client is dependent on you for care, it may be that she is hesitant in asking you to do this for her. However, facial hair can be a source of embarrassment and its removal can greatly improve well-being and confidence. Carers should approach this issue with sensitivity.

In some Western cultures body hair can be considered unattractive and therefore hair from the underarms, legs or pubic area is removed. Some religious groups have requirements to shave specific areas, for example some orthodox Jewish women may shave their heads and always wear wigs. Unless contraindicated on medical grounds, clients should be allowed to follow their usual routines.

Shaving prior to surgical operation

Some surgeons require skin preparation of the area where the incision will be made. This may include shaving of the skin area, which is to prevent infection. Body hair can be removed by wet or dry shaving, but the most important aspect is not to damage the skin. However there is nowadays a growing trend not to shave for *every* surgical operation; it is not now thought to be as necessary as in the past.

Cosmetics

These are preparations which cleanse, beautify or alter appearance. Such items have been used since earliest times by both men and women. However, in western society make-up is not generally worn by men.

Make-up is an important part of body image and carers should encourage clients to maintain their normal appearance as much as possible. For some clients cosmetics may be used as a camouflage to hide a blemish of the skin, for example a severe burn, scar tissue or a birthmark.

Deodorants

These are substances which lessen offensive odours. They act by preventing the growth of bacteria which cause that distinctive body smell. Food we eat can also affect body odour as the smell is excreted by the skin in sweat, for example garlic. Anti-perspirants act by reducing the activity of sweat glands in the skin, thus helping also to reduce odour.

Infestation

It is easy to stand pain, but difficult to stand an itch.

Chang Chao, 1676, from the *Importance of Living*

The very thought of infestation is enough to make you itch. By the time you have read this section it is likely that you will find yourself scratching imaginary insects! But it is an important subject to consider in connection with work as a carer.

Some clients who require assistance with hygiene may be debilitated, suffering from neglect and may also be infested. The invading parasites live by sucking blood from the host after first biting the skin. The constant disturbance of itching and inflammation of the skin causes the client to feel unwell, tired and generally *lousy*.

Attitudes have changed to such parasites. Whereas once they were accepted as a natural part of life to be tolerated, now they are generally regarded with disgust, being largely associated with vagrants, the unkempt and with squalid living conditions. This change in attitude has accompanied the improvement in our standards of living.

It is easy to have negative attitudes towards people who are infested. However, it is important to care for these clients with a sympathetic, caring and non-judgemental approach. Clients should be encouraged to use good personal hygiene to prevent re-infestation. Management and care have to be tactful and realistic, especially if a client is homeless or has a mental health problem. In such circumstances the health team must attempt to solve the underlying problems to promote improvement in the client's overall health.

Lice

There are different types of lice who have adapted to living in different regions of the body. They range from 2 to 4 mm in length. The bites from these lice cause intense itching.

Head lice

These need to gain easy access to the scalp and prefer clean hair, especially the fine hair of children. The close contact of play helps the lice spread from child to child, but they have difficulty in attaching to thick wiry hair and are therefore seldom found in black children.

Lice lay eggs on hair next to the scalp, close to the food supply. The eggs are pale and waxy, about 1 mm long, and can be seen with the naked eye. The eggs (nits) are stuck firmly to the hair and cannot be removed by washing with ordinary shampoo. They can be removed by:

(1) Parting the hair and combing outwards from the hair root using a fine tooth comb
(2) Washing with special shampoos or applying a lotion or oil to detach the nits

Head lice in children are common and spread quickly. Parents are often embarrassed or angry to discover that their child has nits. If one child in a family is affected all the children should be treated or reinfestation is likely to occur.

Body lice

These are much less hardy, being unable to cope with the changes of body temperature. They do not live on the body but in the fibres and seams of clothing, only going on to the skin for sustenance. They live on people who wear the same clothes continuously and who do not take them off to wash.

Body lice can be treated by:

(1) Insecticide powders and sprays
(2) Bathing
(3) Removal and incineration of affected clothes

When dealing with an infested client, wear protective clothing – plastic aprons and gloves. Good standards of personal hygiene and changing and laundering of carers' working clothing make it very unlikely that they will acquire the lice.

Crabs or pubic lice

These prefer coarse hair close to the body as their habitat, normally the pubic region. They have claw-like front feet to cling on to their host and only transfer to another host during sexual contact. They can be treated by the application of special solutions. Sexual partners should be treated at the same time.

Fleas

Human fleas were very common in the past. Men used to shave their heads and wear wigs to reduce infestation. Fleas were also used for purposes of entertainment – flea circuses were once commonplace. Nowadays people are more likely to be bitten by fleas from a dog or cat. If this happens, both the animal and any soft furnishings it has been near or on should be treated. Careful vacuuming of the carpet, especially round the wall, will remove eggs from carpet fibres. Fleas need to be squashed between two hard surfaces to destroy them.

Scabies

Scabies are mites about 0.5 mm long. They burrow under the skin causing red swellings and sometimes a characteristic thin line like a scratch can be seen. Irritation is intense and scratching damages the skin, opening it to infection. Lesions are seen on the hands, between the webs of the fingers. Treatment is by application of solutions to the affected areas.

Summary

Hygiene is a large subject area which has many ramifications for carers. Hygiene is a very personal matter and brings carers into close contact with those for whom they care. Personal choice and rights of the client must always be of paramount importance, care and assistance being offered and given in a tactful and sensitive way.

References

Gooch, J. (1989) Skin hygiene. *Professional Nurse*, **5**(1), 13– 18.

Kahn, R. (1986) Renewing the commitment to oral hygiene. *Geriatric Nursing*, September/October, **7**(5), 244–7.

Further reading

Local organizational policies and procedures

Boyle, S. (1992) Assessing mouth care. *Nursing Times*, 8 April, **88**(15), 44–6.

Greaves, A. (1985) We'll just freshen you up dear. *Nursing Times*, 6 March, **81**(10), 3–4.

Henderson, V. & Nite, G. (1978) *Principles and Practices of Nursing*, 6th edn. Macmillan, Basingstoke.

McMahon, R. (1991) The prevalence of skin problems beneath the breasts of in-patients. *Nursing Times*, 25 September, **87**(39), 48–51.

Millinson, K. (1991) Taking care of John's mouth. *Nursing Times*, 22 May, **87**(21), 34.

Parrot. A. (1991) Teaching mouth care. *Nursing Times*, 18 September, **87**(38), 48.

Roper, N., Logan, W. & Tierney, A. (1990) *The Elements of Nursing*, 3rd ed. Churchill Livingstone, Edinburgh.

Watson, M. (1984) Salt in the bath. *Nursing Times*, November, Occasional Paper (19), 57–9; **80**(46), 14–20.

Wesley-Alexander, J. & Palmquist, J. (1983) The influence of hair-removal methods on wound healing. *Arch. Surgery*, **118**, March.

Williams, K. (1991) *A Practical Approach to Caring*, Chapter 17. Pitman, London.

Chapter 9
Meeting the Nutritional Needs of the Client
Jane Powell with Katie Cullinan

Overview

This chapter takes a close look at food. Food is very important to all of us. Not only is a good diet essential for health but it also plays a major role in other areas of our lives. Think of the role of food at different festive occasions such as Christmas, birthdays and weddings or the role of food as a source of comfort when we feel depressed or unhappy. In this chapter we will try to answer the questions:

- What is a healthy diet?
- What is an appropriate diet for clients with special needs?

- What factors influence our clients' choice of food?

Everyone has their own ideas about food and will have their own likes and dislikes. Try to remember this when thinking about your client's diet and try *not* to allow your own *personal* preferences to influence what your client wishes to eat.

Key words

Healthy diet, nutritional targets, menu planning, swallowing, choking, posture, observation, obesity, diabetes, weight loss, heart disease, constipation, environment, food choice, clients' preferences, timing, eating habits, religious beliefs, vegetarianism.

What is a healthy diet?

Activity 9.1 ■

Before reading any further ask yourself the question: Do I really eat a healthy diet? Do you think your diet is:

- Very healthy?
- Not at all healthy?

- Generally good?

■ ■

The nutritional needs of people change with their age. There are different sets of *healthy eating guidelines* for each of the following age groups:

(1) 0–5 years
(2) 5 years and above
(3) The frail elderly

Healthy eating guidelines for the 0–5 year age group

The set of guidelines for this age group is out of the scope of this chapter (see Further reading).

Activity 9.2 ■

Try to find out about the food and nutrition policy for this group from your local authority or district health authority.

■ ■

Healthy eating guidelines for the 5 years and above age group

According to the Department of Health (1991), the healthy eating guidelines for this age group are:

■ Reduce fat   ■ Reduce sugar
■ Reduce salt   ■ Increase fibre

Reduce fat

Fat contains a lot of calories and is present in many foods. There are two types of fat: *saturated* and *unsaturated*.
   Saturated fats are mainly animal fats and sources include:

■ Meat: beef, pork, lamb, lard,   ■ Fats/oils: coconut oil, palm oil,
   dripping, poultry fat   unspecified vegetable oil, hard
■ Dairy products: full-fat milk,   margarines
   cream, cheese, butter

   Unsaturated fats, including polyunsaturated fats, are oils from vegetables and fatty fish and sources include:

■ Fatty fish: mackerel, herring,   ■ Oils: sunflower, corn, soya,
   salmon, trout, tuna   olive
■ Margarines: sunflower and
   other polyunsaturated ones

There are two main problems associated with eating too much fat:

(1) Fat is loaded with calories. If eaten in too great a quantity it can lead to weight gain and obesity.
(2) Too much saturated fat is linked to an increased risk of heart disease.

The general healthy eating guideline is therefore to cut down on the total amount of fat eaten; use an unsaturated fat in preference to a saturated fat.

Reduce sugar

Sugar is high in calories. Too much sugary food can lead to weight gain and obesity and promotes tooth decay. For these reasons sugary food intake should be reduced.

Sugar gives empty calories, that is it provides energy but no other nutrients such as vitamins, minerals, fibre or protein. If a person has a high intake of sugary foods instead of more nourishing foods their diet may become deficient in essential nutrients.

Sugary foods taste good but are not filling, so it is easy to eat a lot of them. The general healthy eating guideline is to cut down on the amount of sugary foods eaten, especially between meals when they can cause most harm to teeth. Sources of sugar include:

- Sugar, glucose, honey, dextrose, fructose
- Sweets and chocolates
- Sweet desserts and puddings
- Sugary drinks, e.g. fizzy drinks and squash
- Sweet biscuits and cakes
- Sugary breakfast cereals

Reduce salt

On average, we eat ten times more salt per day than our bodies need. Half of this salt comes from processed food such as crisps, ham and other salty meats, gravies and stock cubes, sauces, savoury biscuits, foods in brine, etc. A large proportion of salt is also added to food in cooking and at the table.

For some people eating too much salt can lead to high blood pressure, which in turn can cause heart disease and strokes. To try to prevent this the general guideline is to reduce the amount of salty processed food eaten and cut down on the amount of salt added to food during cooking and at meal times.

Increase fibre

One of the things we should all be eating more of is dietary fibre. Fibre is found in the plant material which we are able to digest. Dietary fibre provides bulk in the diet which gives a feeling of fullness, and because it contains few calories it can help people to control their weight. Research

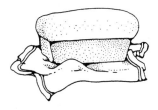

Fig. 9.1 Good sources of dietary fibre.

has suggested that dietary fibre protects against cancer of the bowel, and certain types of dietary fibre can help reduce blood cholesterol levels. When dietary fibre is eaten it absorbs water and softens the stools in the gut, making them easier to pass. Therefore it helps to prevent constipation, diverticular disease and haemorrhoids and can help relieve the pain from haemorrhoids which are already present.

Good sources of dietary fibre include:

- Wholemeal or high bran breads.
- Wholegrain or bran-enriched breakfast cereals, e.g. Allbran, Branflakes, Weetabix, Shredded Wheat.
- Foods made with wholemeal flour.
- Fruits of all kinds especially if skin is eaten; dried fruit, prunes, apricots and bananas are particularly good.
- Vegetables of all kinds, especially peas, beans and lentils.
- Wholemeal pasta, brown rice.

Note:

When high fibre foods are eaten it is very important that plenty of fluids are taken during the day. At least eight cups of fluid should be drunk (*see* Fig. 9.3), for example water, fruit juice, squash, milk, tea, coffee.

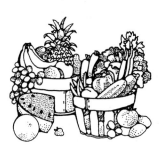

Fig. 9.2 Good sources of dietary fibre.

Alcohol

Large quantities of alcohol should be avoided as it can damage the body, especially the liver. Alcoholic drinks contain a lot of calories so can cause weight gain. If obesity is a problem, alcohol should be avoided. Low calorie drinks can be used as a substitute.

The safe limits for alcohol are 14 units per week for women and 21 units per week for men. (One unit is either half a pint of ordinary beer, one measure of spirit or a standard glass of wine.)

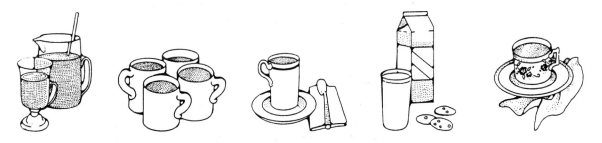

Fig. 9.3 Drink at least eight cups of fluid daily when eating a high fibre diet.

Activity 9.3 ■

Compare your own diet with the healthy eating guidelines. Do you eat a healthy diet? If you feel that your diet could be improved, make a list of the changes you need to make.

■ ■

Healthy eating guidelines for the frail elderly

Food is essential for both physical and social well-being whatever a person's age. However for frail elderly people it is often more important to ensure that they are getting adequate nutrition than to be overzealous in encouraging them to follow the Department of Health (1992) healthy eating guidelines.

Activity 9.4 ■

Which of the healthy eating guidelines for the 5 years and above age group apply to frail elderly people?

■ ■

Fat intake

For the frail elderly, fat should only be reduced if the client is overweight. Fat is a valuable source of vitamins A and D, which are essential to maintain good health. People often want to eat less as they become older, therefore fat in the diet can become a useful source of energy. Although the frail elderly do not need to reduce the normal amount of fat in their diets it is not advisable for them to eat excessive amounts of fatty foods.

Sugar intake

Clients in the frail elderly age group should only cut down their sugar intake if they are trying to lose weight, are diabetic or still have their own teeth. The sections on weight reduction and diabetes will explain why sugar should be reduced in these two situations. If a client has a poor appetite, sugar is a very useful source of energy.

Salt intake

Older people have fewer taste buds than when they were young so cannot taste foods as well as they used to. An unnecessarily severe salt restriction should not be encouraged as it can make food less palatable and less interesting. This will affect the client's desire to eat.

Fibre intake

Fibre in the diet should be increased. Older people are more likely than younger ones to suffer from constipation, and it can be a very common problem in this age group. When high fibre foods are eaten it is essential that plenty of fluids are taken throughout the day. This may be more difficult for older people who tend to have a reduced sense of thirst and who may suffer from and worry about incontinence, especially at night. Drinks can be taken earlier in the day to help overcome this problem.

What about vitamins and minerals?

A good dietary supply of vitamins and minerals is essential. If your client is eating a well-balanced diet with plenty of variety and in appropriate quantities it is likely that they are getting all the vitamins and minerals they need. However, if they have a poor diet or poor appetite, or if they have increased dietary needs due to a medical condition, it may be necessary for your client to take a vitamin supplement. Table 9.1 lists sources of important vitamins and minerals.

Table 9.1 Sources of important vitamins and minerals.

Vitamin B complex		
Vitamin B1 (thiamin)	Wholegrain cereals, nuts, meat, fish, pulses, yeast extract.	Helps in the breakdown of foods to provide energy.
Vitamin B2 (riboflavin)	Liver, milk, eggs.	
Nicotinic acid	Wholegrain cereals, meat, fish, liver, pulses.	Used by nervous system.
Folic acid and vitamin B12	Liver, green vegetables, meat, eggs, yeast extract.	Blood formation; prevents anaemia.
Vitamin D	Oily fish (e.g. herring, sardines, pilchards), eggs, margarines, yoghurt, evaporated milk and breakfast cereals.	Helps to keep bones healthy.
Calcium	Cheese, milk, yoghurt, fish, pulses, dark green vegetables.	With vitamin D it helps to keep bones and teeth healthy and strong.
Vitamin C	Citrus fruits and their juices, vitamin C enriched squash, blackcurrant squash, green vegetables, potatoes.	Aids iron absorption; helps body to fight infection and heals wounds.
Iron	Liver, kidney, red meat, wholemeal bread, dried fruit.	Blood formation; prevents anaemia.

Menu planning

When planning a menu for a client there are many factors to take into consideration. Whenever possible the client should be encouraged to take part in planning their own menu. As a carer you can help, encourage,

Table 9.2 Daily nutritional targets.

Food	Quantity	Comments
Milk	$\frac{1}{2}$–1 pint per day.	Use on cereals, in puddings and drinks, yoghurt or cheese can be a useful source of calcium, as are fish, whose bones are eaten.
	Two portions from this list daily.	
Meat Fish	60–90 g 120–150 g } cooked weights	Liver, red meats, corned beef are useful sources of iron; oily fish provide vitamin D.
Cheese	60 g	
Eggs	2	
Pulses (beans and peas)	60 g dried weight	Use pulses in soups, casseroles or salads.
Bread Breakfast cereal Pasta Rice Potatoes	At least one portion at each meal.	Use jacket potatoes, wholemeal bread and pasta and brown rice to increase the fibre content.
Vegetables: fresh or frozen Salad	Two portions per day.	These provide fibre, vitamins and minerals.
Fruit: fresh, stewed, tinned or dried Fruit juice	One portion per day.	Try to include citrus fruit two or three times each week.
Fluids	*At least* eight cups of fluid per day.	For example water, squash, fruit juice, milk, tea, coffee; this helps to prevent constipation and maintain health.

advise and support your client in planning their menu, but your client must have the final say in choosing the foods they wish to eat.

When planning a menu try to ensure that:

(1) The client's individual food preferences have been taken into account.
(2) The nutritional recommendations have been met (see Table 9.2) and nutritional deficiencies do not arise.
(3) Any special dietary needs have been taken into account.
(4) A wide variety of foods and cooking methods have been used.
(5) A sufficient variety of colour, taste and texture has been included in the meals.
(6) The food items on the menu are readily available.
(7) The right cooking equipment is available.
(8) The meal is within the budget of the client or catering department.
(9) The meal is served at the appropriate time for the client.
(10) The cooking practices are within the current food hygiene regulations (Foodsense, 1992).

This may sound very complicated but most of us are already doing it for ourselves and families. However, we cannot use our own personal preferences to plan a meal for our clients. *It is essential that a client's own food preferences and needs are recognized and are respected.*

Daily nutritional needs

To help ensure that nutritional recommendations are met, *minimum daily nutritional targets* can be used to plan a menu (see Table 9.2). It must be stressed that these are minimum amounts of food to be taken each day; the actual amounts needed for an individual will vary according to age, sex and activity levels.

Monitoring your client's food and drink intake

There are two main situations when you may be asked to monitor a client's food and drink intake.

(1) To check that a client is eating the correct quantity and type of food;
(2) To check that a client is having the right quantity of fluid.

The easiest way to monitor a client's food and drink intake is via a food record chart; an example of a chart is shown in Table 9.3. The quantity and type of food eaten should be recorded as accurately as possible. For instance, if a client eats a sandwich you should record how many slices of bread were eaten, whether it was white or wholemeal, the sandwich filling, and whether all of it was eaten. Remember to write down what was actually eaten or drunk rather than what was served. The more accurate the description of the food, the more useful it will be.

Table 9.3 Food record chart.

Date	Write down type and quantity of food and drink taken
Breakfast	
Mid-morning	
Lunch	
Mid-afternoon	
Supper	
Bedtime	
Daily foods, e.g. milk	
Other foods	

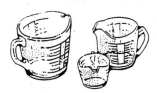

Fig. 9.4 Measuring fluids.

The quantity of food and drink can be written either as household measures (e.g. a bowl, half a cup, a full mug, two slices of meat, etc.) or it may need to be recorded more accurately (e.g. 150 ml tea, 90 ml soup, (see Fig. 9.4) 50 g meat, 120 g potato). If you measure quantities of food and drink every day you will soon become familiar with how much certain cups, bowls, mugs and plates hold. If a client is not meeting their daily target for food or drink it is important to notify the appropriate member of the health care team as soon as possible.

Activity 9.5 ■

Complete your own food record chart for one day. Do not miss out any food or drink and accurately record the quantities eaten. Compare your food and fluid intake to the daily nutritional targets (see Table 9.2). Are you having the right quantities of food and drink?

■ ■

Swallowing and swallowing difficulties

Normal swallowing process

When you eat and drink you do so without thinking. However, if something goes wrong (for example if you have an anaesthetic injection at the dentist, you may dribble when you drink) you soon realize how important it is to have your face and mouth in full working order so you can eat and drink comfortably.

For *normal swallowing* to take place your cheeks, lips, tongue, soft palate and muscles in the throat and those going down to the stomach need to work properly. Normal swallowing can be divided into three main stages involving:

(1)   The mouth (oral stage)
(2)   The throat (pharyngeal stage)
(3)   The tube leading from the throat to the stomach (oesophageal stage)

Oral stage

This is the only part of swallowing of which you are consciously aware. When you take a bite of food you chew it and move it round in your mouth, mixing it with saliva until it is soft enough to swallow. You make the food into a ball (bolus) in the middle of your mouth with your tongue and cheeks (Fig. 9.5(a)), push it to the back of your mouth with your tongue and the reflex part of swallowing begins (Fig. 9.5(b)). With a sip of drink it is similar, only you don't chew it but form a bolus straight away.

Pharyngeal stage

Once the swallowing reflex is triggered everything is automatic and you cannot interrupt the process. The soft palate at the back of the mouth raises up so that food or drink cannot get up your nose and the bolus is squeezed into the throat. At the same time your voice box moves up to help push the food or drink further down your throat (Fig. 9.5(c)). The vocal cords in the voice box are closed and the epiglottis folds down over the entrance to the windpipe (trachea) to stop the food or liquid going down the wrong way into your lungs (Fig. 9.5(d)).

Oesophageal stage

The bolus is squeezed the whole length of the oesophagus by muscles contracting in waves (peristalsis) until it reaches the stomach (Fig. 9.5(e)). Swallowing is now finished and digestion begins.

?

Did you know?

Did you know that you swallow automatically on average 600 times over a 24 hour period?

Activity 9.6   ■

List the factors which might influence swallowing.

Your list may include:

■ taste	■ smell of food
■ appetite	■ sight
■ texture of food	■ anxiety
■ illness	■ age
■ state of mouth	■ mood
■ food preferences	■ culture
■ being fed	

■ ■

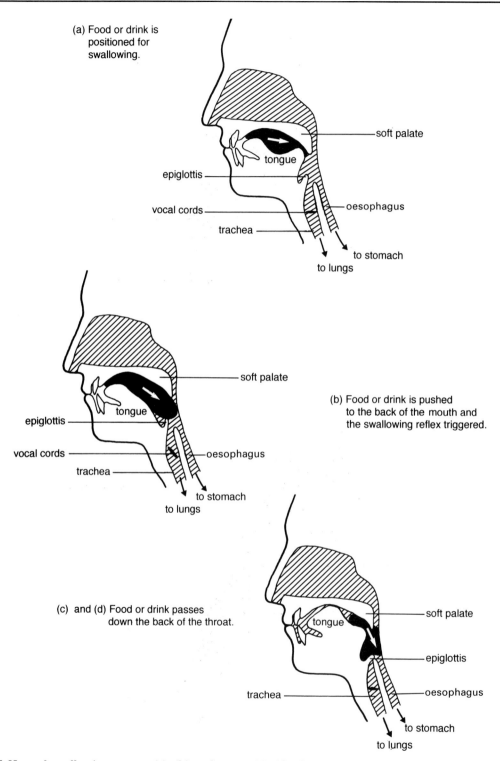

Fig. 9.5 Normal swallowing stages: (a), (b) oral stage; (c), (d) pharyngeal stage; (e) oesophageal stage.

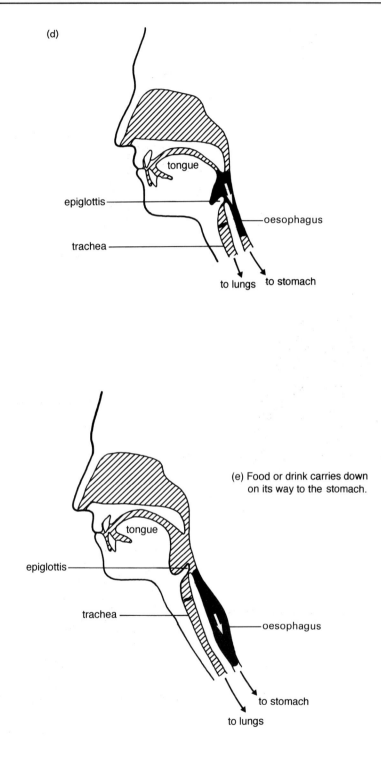

(d)

tongue

epiglottis

oesophagus

trachea

to lungs   to stomach

(e) Food or drink carries down
on its way to the stomach.

tongue

epiglottis

trachea

oesophagus

to stomach

to lungs

What causes swallowing difficulties

Swallowing difficulties (dysphagia) can be caused by a variety of disorders ranging from stroke, Parkinson's disease, multiple sclerosis and head injury to laryngectomy (removal of the voice box).

What happens in dysphagia?

In the mouth

You may notice that your client is drooling or having difficulty chewing or moving food around the mouth. They may not be able to clear food from the sides of the mouth. This is often due to poor control of the lips, tongue and cheeks and poor sensation in the mouth. Other problems you may notice during this stage are loss of taste and smell.

In the throat

Your client may cough or choke when eating or drinking. This might be because the swallowing reflex is delayed or absent (e.g. after a stroke) so the food or drink trickles down the back of the throat into the wind pipe (trachea). Because the automatic part of swallowing has not been started the epiglottis has not folded down and the vocal cords are not shut. This process of food or liquid going down the wrong way and entering the wind pipe is called *aspiration*. It is potentially very dangerous as the lungs are designed for air, so if food or drink get in, a chest infection is likely to develop and cause breathing complications.

In the oesophagus

It is difficult to observe problems during this stage, but clients may complain of discomfort in their chest just after they swallow.

Care required for clients with swallowing difficulties

When you are with a client who has swallowing difficulties you can help in a number of ways.

(1)   Observation

■   What helps your client to swallow? For example:
      soft food;
      cold food.
■   Which foods does your client find more difficult to swallow?

(2)   Posture

■   Look at how your client is sitting. Posture should be as upright as possible so that food is helped to go down the right way (Figs 9.6 and 9.7).

Fig. 9.6 Posture.

Fig. 9.7 Posture.

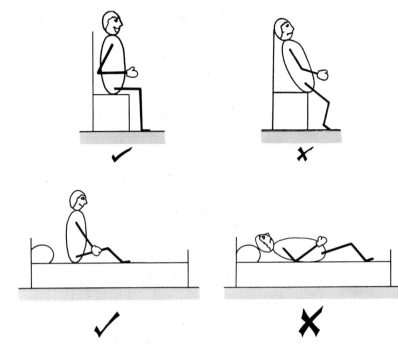

(3)   Consistency of food and drink

■   Think about the different textures and consistencies of food (e.g. soft food may be easier to swallow than hard food which requires a lot of chewing). If clients require food of a specific consistency make their diet as interesting as possible and try to use a variety of different foods. Try to ensure that your clients are meeting their daily nutritional targets.

■   When helping your client to eat, give only one consistency at a time in small amounts.

■   Look to see if it is easier to drink through a straw than from a cup.

■   Look to see which liquids are easier to swallow (e.g. thick soup rather than tea). Some clients need to have all their drinks thickened. There are several thickening agents available; some will be more suited to your client than others.

■   Contact your local speech and language therapist or dietitian for further information on a specific client's individual needs.

■   Notify the client's doctor or dietitian if your client is having problems with their diet or if they are losing weight.

(4)   Timing

■   Allow plenty of time when your clients eat. Let them dictate the pace.

(5)   Temperature

■   In general, cold liquids and food are easier to swallow than hot.

Remember that being fed is rarely a pleasant experience, so try to make it as agreeable as possible by doing things the way your client likes. Always ask advice from members of the team involved in the care of clients with swallowing difficulties before helping them to eat or drink. In particular, consult the speech and language therapist, the dietitian and physiotherapist.

Activity 9.7 ■■■■■■■■■■■■■■■■■■■■■■■■■■■■■■

 Get a dry biscuit and a cup of water. Have a bit of biscuit – bend your head to the side – now try to swallow. Have a sip of water – try to swallow with your mouth open. Give someone else something to eat or drink. Ask someone to feed you. How does it feel?

■■■■■■■■■■■■■■■■■■■■■■■■■■■■■■■■

How to deal with a choking emergency

Do	*Don't*
Be calm and reassuring. Encourage your client to relax.	Slap your client's back unless the head is lower than the lungs, otherwise the obstruction could move further down, as gravity and inhaled air would encourage this to happen.
Try to remove any visible obstruction from the back of the mouth.	
Encourage your client to lean forward with his/her chin tucked in. If this is not successful call for help.	

Therapeutic diets

In this section we will briefly look at some common therapeutic diets. If you would like more detailed information on these or other therapeutic diets, or you are worried about a particular client following a therapeutic diet, contact the nutrition and dietetic department at your local hospital.

Obesity and the weight-reducing diet

Obesity is a very common nutritional problem. It can lead to disorders such as high blood pressure, diabetes, gallstones, stroke and coronary heart disease and it aggravates arthritis. Obesity occurs when a person eats more energy-giving food than their body needs. This extra energy is then stored as body fat. The principle of a weight-reducing diet is to eat less energy than the body needs so that the body fat stores are used up. However it is still *very* important to have a good daily intake of all the other essential nutrients such as protein, vitamins, minerals and dietary fibre. Clients needing to lose weight for medical reasons should have a personal diet sheet, preferably from a dietitian.

For general weight reduction the following guidelines are used:

(1)   Encourage three meals a day: breakfast, lunch and supper.
(2)   Between-meal snacks should be avoided.
(3)   Fried foods and fatty foods should be avoided.
(4)   Sweet and sugary foods should be avoided.
(5)   Artificial sweeteners and low calorie drinks can be used, but diabetic foods and slimming aids should be avoided.
(6)   Fruit should be encouraged in place of puddings.
(7)   Encourage intake of high fibre foods to help satisfy the appetite.
(8)   All alcoholic drinks should be avoided.
(9)   Weight should be lost slowly and consistently: 1–2 lb a week is ideal.
(10) When possible, exercise should be taken within the individual's own ability.

If a person is very overweight it will take them many months to reach their ideal body weight. During that time it is important to offer them plenty of support and encouragement with their diet.

Weight reduction for older people is particularly difficult as they are often unable to exercise and may only need a relatively small quantity of food each day. Before it is suggested that an older person follows a weight-reducing diet it is important to clarify who will benefit from it. Is it the carers or the client? If it is the carers who will benefit most, the client should not be expected to follow a restricted diet.

Activity 9.8   ■

If you need to lose weight, list the changes you should make to your diet. If you lost 2 lb per week, how long would it take you to reach your target weight?

■ ■

Diabetes and the diabetic diet

Diabetes is a disorder in which the body is unable to control the amount of sugar (i.e. glucose) in the blood. It is essential to have the right amount of sugar in the blood if the body is to function properly.

What happens normally?

Sugar is absorbed from food in the gut into the blood stream. For the body to use this sugar, the pancreas (a gland in the abdomen) produces a hormone called insulin. Insulin allows the sugar in the blood to pass into the tissues of the body where it can be used as energy.

What happens when a person has diabetes?

Diabetes is a condition where the pancreas is unable to produce enough insulin to allow the sugar to move from the blood into the tissues. The sugar is therefore trapped in the blood and, unless treated, its levels will rise uncontrollably.

When the blood sugar level is too high, small amounts of sugar overflow into the urine. This can lead to several problems:

- Sugar will draw water into the urine, making the diabetic person want to pass water frequently through the day and night.
- As this extra water is lost the body becomes dehydrated, causing the person to become extremely thirsty.
- Sugar in the urine is excellent food for bacteria and can lead to urinary infection.

There are also more serious side-effects to diabetes. The likelihood of getting these is increased if the client does not follow the correct diabetic treatment.

Treatment

There are three types of treatment for diabetes:

- Diet alone   ■ Diet and tablets
- Diet and insulin injection

Whatever the form of treatment it is important to remember that the client will always need to follow a diabetic diet. Clients with diabetes should have their own personal dietary advice from a dietitian, diabetes nurse or doctor. It is important that your client's diabetic control is regularly reviewed as treatment often needs to be changed as people become older.

The general dietary guidelines for clients with diabetes are:

(1) Eat regular meals containing starchy foods (e.g. bread, potato, pasta, rice, chapatis).
(2) Do not miss meals.
(3) If recommended by a dietitian, diabetes nurse or doctor it may be necessary to take regular between-meal snacks.
(4) Avoid sweet and sugary food and drink.
(5) If overweight try to lose the extra weight.
(6) Try to eat a wholemeal or high fibre food with each meal.
(7) Do not use diabetic products as they are expensive, not low calorie and some contain a sweetener called sorbitol which can cause diarrhoea. Diabetic squash and jams or marmalade may be taken.
(8) Avoid fat and fatty food (especially if the client is overweight).
(9) Alcohol may be taken in moderation but not on an empty stomach. Sweet alcoholic drinks should be avoided.

These are only general guidelines and you will find that individual dietary advice may vary slightly.

Hypoglycaemia

People who are taking insulin or certain diabetic tablets may be affected by hypoglycaemia (often called a *hypo*). This is when the blood sugar becomes too low. Early warning signs vary from person to person and include shaking, trembling, confusion, sweating, tingling sensations, palpitations and becoming absent-minded or argumentative. Diabetic people usually recognize their own symptoms.

Hypoglycaemia can arise if a client taking insulin or certain diabetic drugs:

- Misses or delays a meal or snack
- Takes strenuous exercise over and above their usual level of exercise
- Does not eat enough starchy food
- Takes more insulin than needed
- Takes too much alcohol

Hypoglycaemia must be treated immediately, if not your client could lose consciousness.

How should hypoglycaemia be treated?

If your client has the above symptoms, try to get them to take a small amount of a sugary food, for example:

- 1 eggcupful of Lucozade (50 ml)
- 3 Dextrosol tablets
- $^3/_4$ cup of ordinary lemonade (150 ml)
- 2 lumps/teaspoon of sugar
- $^1/_2$ cup of ordinary Coke (100 ml)

This should make them feel better within a few minutes, after which they should have:

either 1 cup of milk and a biscuit,
or   2 digestive biscuits,
or   2 slices of bread as a sandwich.

Alternatively if it is time for their next meal they should eat it straight away. If your client frequently suffers from hypos their doctor should be notified.

What if your client becomes ill?

If a diabetic client, taking insulin or diabetic tablets, becomes ill, it is very important that they do not stop taking their medication. This is because illness (e.g. influenza, diarrhoea, colds) will cause a natural rise in blood

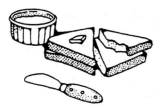

Fig. 9.8 Sandwich.

sugar. Non-diabetic people can cope with this, but people with diabetes must continue taking their medication in order to control it.

It is important for your client to eat regular meals and snacks. If they do not feel like a full meal, encourage them to take frequent snacks through the day, such as soup and bread, milk, yoghurt, sandwiches (Fig. 9.8).

Weight loss and poor appetite

Weight loss occurs when a client has a poor appetite, when nutritional intake is reduced or when illness causes an increased energy requirement, i.e. when more energy is used by the body than is being eaten in the diet. If a client is poorly nourished they should be encouraged to take a high energy, high protein diet in order to meet their nutritional needs.

Appetite can be increased by encouraging small, frequent meals regularly throughout the day and by offering foods which are enjoyable and attractively presented. People need plenty of encouragement to eat if they have a poor appetite but with perseverance their appetite should improve.

High protein foods such as meat, fish, eggs, cheese and milk should be encouraged. Try offering milky drinks instead of tea, coffee or squash. Milk can be made more nutritious by adding two tablespoons of milk powder to one pint of whole milk. This fortified milk can then be used for drinks, cereals, cooking, etc.

Avoid giving large quantities of food as this can often be a turn off for people with a poor appetite.

Dietary supplements are a useful way of adding extra nourishment to the diet. They are products which contain a concentrated source of nourishment in a relatively small quantity. They are usually in the form of drinks or soups and can either be bought from chemists or obtained on prescription for certain medical conditions. Examples include Build-up, Complan and Vitafood (available from a chemist) and Fortisip, Fresubin and Ensure (available on prescription only). If your client has been advised to take a dietary supplement encourage them to take it regularly as advised by their doctor or dietitian.

It should be remembered that a reduction in body weight is only one indicator of a poor diet and only relates to energy intake. Deficiencies of other nutrients can occur whilst body weight remains constant. Skin changes, poor wound healing, anaemia and self neglect may all be indicators of a poor diet. If you feel that your client is at risk of developing nutritional deficiencies, notify your client's doctor, nurse or dietitian.

Eating for a healthy heart

The general healthy eating guidelines for the 5 years and above age group form the basic dietary information for *eating for a healthy heart.* One of the most important factors in *heart disease* is *obesity*. If a client is overweight try to encourage them to lose weight. However, some people may need more specific advice if they are particularly at risk from heart disease.

There are two types of fat in the blood: cholesterol and triglycerides.

A high cholesterol level or a high cholesterol and triglyceride level can increase the risk of heart disease. The type of diet your client will need to follow depends on whether it is only their cholesterol level which is raised or whether their cholesterol and triglyceride levels are raised. Always refer to a client's own personal dietary advice if possible.

Dietary advice for a high cholesterol level

(1) Fats, particularly saturated fats, should be avoided as they tend to increase cholesterol levels.
(2) Unsaturated fats, including polyunsaturated fats, tend to lower cholesterol levels and should be used in moderation instead of saturated fats. The total intake of fat in a client's diet should be reduced and low fat foods should be encouraged.
(3) Cholesterol-rich foods should be limited (e.g. liver, kidney, heart, egg yolk, shellfish).
(4) Dietary fibre is beneficial and should be encouraged as a regular part of the diet.

What if the triglyceride level is also raised?

If a client has a high cholesterol level *and* a high triglyceride level there are two *extra* pieces of advice they should follow.

(1) Alcohol must be strictly limited.
(2) All sweet and sugary food should be avoided and regular amounts of starchy food taken through the day. Sugar and starchy food will affect the level of triglycerides in the blood.

Factors influencing food choice

There are many factors that influence food choice. These include religious beliefs and cultural influences in addition to physical, psychological, environmental and social factors.

Religious beliefs affecting food choice

In most religions there are rules or conventions about food. These are used as one of the expressions of orthodoxy and unity between members of a faith. It is important to clarify with the individual client what they do and do not eat. Some of the religious rules about food and drink are shown below.

Hindu

■ Most Hindus will not eat meat or fish of any kind. Less strict Hindus may eat lamb, chicken or white fish. It is most unusual for Hindus to eat beef or pork.

- Very strict Hindus may not eat eggs since they are potentially a source of life.
- Animal fats such as dripping, lard and some margarines are not acceptable. Ghee (clarified butter) and vegetable oils are used in cooking.
- Strict Hindus will be unwilling to eat food unless they are certain that the utensils used in the preparation and serving of food are not in contact with meat or fish.
- Some Hindus fast for one or two days a week. This is sometimes for specific reasons. Fasting may involve missing one or more meals a day or abstinence from everything except dairy produce or fruit and nuts all day.

Muslim

- Pork and all products of pigs or any carnivorous animals are forbidden.
- All meat should be ritually slaughtered (Halal); kosher meat may be acceptable.
- Alcohol, including that used in cooking, is forbidden.
- All healthy adult Muslims are expected to fast for the 30 days of Ramadan. For the whole month they are not permitted to eat or drink from dawn to dusk.

Sikh

- Some Sikhs, especially women, are vegetarian but many eat chicken, lamb and fish.
- They are unlikely to eat beef or pork.

Jewish

- Pork and all products of the pig are forbidden.
- Fish with scales and fins are allowed, shellfish are not.
- Meat and milk must not be served at the same meal or cooked together.
- All meat and poultry must be kosher, i.e. it must undergo a ritual method of slaughter.

Rastafarian

- They are forbidden to eat pork and all vine products, e.g. currants, raisins, grapes and wine.
- Most are vegetarian or vegan. Some Rastafarians will eat fish.
- Processed foods and additives are avoided as much as possible.
- Frozen food is acceptable, but canned or tinned foods are not.
- Wholemeal foods are considered especially beneficial and are preferred to refined products.
- Alcohol is not permitted.

Seventh Day Adventists

- They do not eat pork or pork products.
- Many devout Adventists are vegetarians.
- They may fast at certain times – for instance, they may give up rich or sweet foods during Lent.

Cultural influences

Traditional foods vary from one culture to another and have developed over many years. They are largely based on the plants most suitable for that particular region and on the wildlife or domesticated animals available. For instance Ireland has a climate particularly suited to growing potatoes whilst many parts of Asia and Africa have soils and a climate suited to growing rice.

In recent years, foods have become widely available from all regions of the world. It is unnecessary for people from other countries and cultures living in Britain to change to traditional British foods. If you are caring for a client who prefers to eat their own culture's traditional foods, every effort should be made to make these foods available to them.

Diets based on personal ethics and beliefs

Vegetarian and vegan diets

Vegetarians do not eat meat and poultry and some do not eat fish, eggs or dairy products. The degree to which a person follows a vegetarian diet depends on the individual and is usually based on religious or moral beliefs. Vegans do not eat any animal products, i.e. meat, fish, eggs or dairy products.

Meat and other animal products are a rich source of protein in the diet. Vegetarians and vegans use other sources of protein such as pulses (beans and peas) and their products (e.g. soya milk and tofu) and nuts. However, nutritional deficiencies can occur if a person stops eating animal products and does not replace them with an alternative source of nutrients.

If your client follows a vegetarian or vegan diet, find out exactly what foods are eaten and how the client prefers them to be cooked.

A vegetarian or vegan diet can be a very healthy way of eating and should include a wide variety of foods to provide the essential nutrients. There are many books available on vegetarian and vegan diets. If you are unsure how to cater for vegans or vegetarians, talk to your client, refer to recipe books or contact your local dietitian.

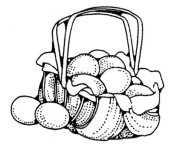

Fig. 9.9 Free-range eggs.

Activity 9.9 ■

Try to plan a one-day menu for someone following a vegetarian diet, who does not eat meat/fish/eggs. Look at the nutritional targets earlier in the chapter to ensure that you have provided the correct number of servings from each of the food groups.

■ ■

Other diets based on personal preference

Some people follow diets based on personal preferences. For instance, it is becoming increasingly common for people to choose organic foods or free-range animal products (Fig. 9.9). If a client prefers to eat particular foods based on *personal preference*, *religious beliefs* or *moral grounds* their wishes must be respected and every effort made to accommodate their needs.

Physical and mental factors affecting food choice

There are many physical and psychological factors that can affect food choice.

Poor dentition and chewing difficulties

A client's ability to chew food will be reduced if they have severe tooth decay, poorly fitting dentures, sore or infected gums, mouth ulcers or if they have no teeth or dentures at all. Clients should be encouraged to eat food which can be chewed properly and which contains all the essential nutrients. If clients need to wear dentures ensure that they are in place before the meal is served. Try to encourage your clients to have regular dental treatment.

Swallowing difficulties

Refer to the section on swallowing and swallowing difficulties. Choking on food or drink can be extremely unpleasant and off-putting. If your client has a swallowing problem, give them plenty of support and encouragement to eat and drink a sufficient quantity to achieve their daily nutritional targets.

Taste and smell

The taste and smell of food influences our desire to eat it. If a client's perception of taste or smell changes, foods which were once appealing can seem bland and tasteless or even sour and metallic. Changes in taste and smell perception can occur for several reasons including stroke, drugs, chemotherapy and radiotherapy. Taste and smell perception also diminishes with age – you often hear old people say that 'food doesn't taste like it used to'. Talk to your clients to find out which foods taste best and avoid

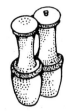

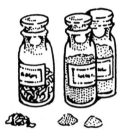

Fig. 9.10 Condiments and spices.

giving them food which they find unpleasant. Adding flavourings to food can improve taste, e.g. pepper, vinegar, salt, mustard, sugar (see Fig. 9.10).

Communication difficulties

Good communication with a client is essential if the client is to make their own informed choice of food and drink. Speech, language, hearing difficulties and poor eyesight can affect communication not only between carer and client, but also with other people involved with the provision of food, e.g. milkman, shop assistants, meals-on-wheels service, etc. Every effort should be made to communicate clearly with the client and for the client to express their wishes and needs regarding food and drink.

Poor vision

Well presented and attractive looking food can influence food choice. If your client is unable to see they will not gain any stimulation from the food's appearance. Poor vision will also affect your client's ability to read food labels, sell-by dates, cooking instructions, etc. If your client needs assistance with eating and drinking, describe the food to them and where it is situated on their plate. Eating and drinking aids may be useful to these clients.

Physical disabilities

Some clients may experience physical difficulty with eating, drinking, shopping or cooking. If your client has eating and drinking aids encourage their use and encourage your client to maintain their independence. The occupational therapist can help the client by adapting their environment or advising on the use of various types of eating and drinking aids (Fig. 9.11).

Breathing difficulties

Shortness of breath and other breathing problems can affect a client's food intake. To swallow food or drink it is necessary to momentarily stop breathing. People who have a breathing problem can therefore find it difficult to eat much at any one time. To overcome this, food and drink should be offered in small quantities frequently throughout the day. High calorie foods or dietary supplements may be advised if the client is losing weight.

Constipation and incontinence

Constipation can cause the feeling of fullness, nausea and general distress. Clients who are constipated may have a reduced appetite. To help resolve the constipation encourage them to eat high fibre foods with plenty to drink.

Fig. 9.11 Aids for eating for a client with rheumatoid arthritis.

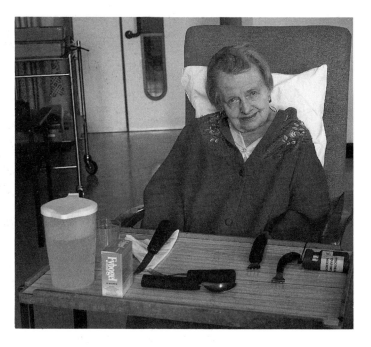

The fear of urinary incontinence may result in clients only wanting to drink very small quantities of fluid. Incontinence at night can be reduced by drinking more in the morning and less in the late afternoon and evening.

Drugs

There are many drugs whose side-effects interfere with food intake. This may affect your client by causing taste changes, nausea, diarrhoea or constipation and reduced ability to absorb nutrients from food. If you notice these side-effects when your client starts a new drug, notify the appropriate member of the health care team.

Mental health problems

Dementia, confusion, depression and anxiety can all result in a change in nutritional intake. Communication with the client may be difficult and they may not be able to express their food preferences or needs. Some people with mental health problems have altered dietary requirements, e.g. hyperactivity will result in an increase in nutritional needs.

Environmental and social factors affecting food choice

The food choice available, the way a meal is served and the environment a client is expected to eat in will all influence the client's nutritional intake (Fig. 9.12).

Fig. 9.12 Serving lunch.

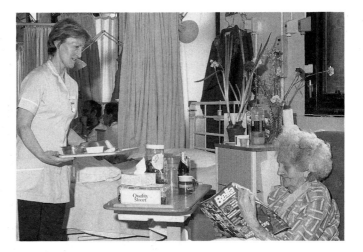

Activity 9.10 ■

How do you prefer to eat your meals? Do you prefer to:

- Eat alone or with others?
- Sit at a table or eat from a tray on your lap?
- Watch television while eating, sit quietly or chat with others?
- Use a favourite dish, glass or cutlery?
- Eat your meal quickly or take a long time to eat, with a break between your main course and pudding?
- Have your food presented in a particular way?
- Have control over the amount of food served on your plate, having larger helpings of the foods you particularly like?

■ ■

We all like to have some control over the food we eat. This control can be lost when food is prepared or served by others. An individual's needs and wishes must be acknowledged if they are to get the most benefit out of meal times.

Activity 9.11 ■

The following list shows some of the ways meal times can be made more pleasant for clients. Tick those that you feel you are already doing. Put a cross next to the ones you need to pay more attention to.

- Encourage clients to do as much as possible for themselves.
- Serve food at a time preferred by the client.
- Allow clients to eat at their own pace. Never hurry them to finish.
- When necessary, help your client to move to the area they wish to eat in.

- Help your client to obtain a safe and comfortable position for eating and drinking.
- Ask your client if they wish to go to the toilet and wash their hands before and after eating. When necessary help them to achieve this.
- If necessary, help your client to wipe away excess food from their face, hands and clothing during and after a meal. Do this in a way which does not cause them to lose their dignity.
- If your client would like to be provided with protection for their clothes such as an apron or a serviette, help them to position it so that they do not lose their dignity, and their food intake is not restricted.
- When possible, clients should have freedom about where and with whom they sit.
- Try to ensure that the environment for eating is pleasant and accommodates the wishes of the client.
- When possible, use tablecloths, serviettes, and attractive crockery and cutlery (Fig. 9.13).
- Remove unnecessary items from the area the client wishes to eat in, e.g. Zimmer frames, commodes, nursing or medical notes, urine bottles, etc.
- Meal times may be the highlight of the day for many clients. Try to make meals an enjoyable social occasion.
- The choice of food available should be well displayed or explained clearly to your clients.
- Ensure that personal taste preferences are known and catered for.
- Encourage clients to choose the most suitable and appropriate options, and when asked explain the reasons for this. Give clients the final say in choosing the food *they* wish to eat.
- If your client dislikes the food offered provide a suitable alternative.
- Serve food in sensible portion sizes or as the client needs or wishes.
- Try to ensure that the presentation, consistency and temperature of the food and drink served are as the client needs or wishes.
- When possible, offer the client second helpings at meal times.
- Provide a range of condiments which are within easy reach of your client, e.g. salt, pepper, pickles, relishes, mustard, horseradish, etc. (Fig. 9.14).
- When possible, encourage your client to serve themselves or, if eating in a communal setting, to serve others.
- If possible, food should be served as it would be in an individual's home, i.e. serving dishes placed on the table, meat carved at the table, etc.
- Ensure that food is placed within easy reach of the client.
- Encourage social contact at meal times between clients or carer and client.
- Help your client to eat in a socially acceptable manner.
- In a communal setting provide appropriate seating arrangements for clients with anti-social eating habits.
- Having to be fed often feels undignified. Respect your client's dignity and help them to do as much as possible for themselves.

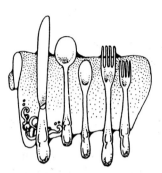

Fig. 9.13 Favourite cutlery and serviette.

Fig. 9.14 Offer a range of condiments.

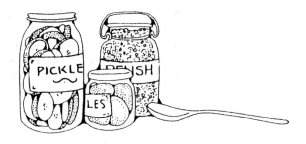

- Ensure that any eating or drinking aids are used properly.
- Avoid interrupting the client during meal times.
- Clear up well after a meal and dispose of left-over food safely.
- Ensure that the client is offered and has easy access to suitable and enjoyable food and drink between meals.
- Follow the current food hygiene regulations when dealing with food and drink (refer to Chapter 6).
- Eating is a fundamental part of our daily lives. A carer's positive attitude to helping clients with eating and drinking will increase the likelihood of their client achieving a good nutritional intake.

Summary

- An adequate and appropriate intake of food and drink is essential for your client's general good health.
- Be familiar with your client's normal eating habits. You may be the first person to notice a change.
- Always discuss your client's dietary problems with an appropriate member of the health care team.
- Obtain the agreement of your supervisor and of the client when suggesting changes to your client's diet.
- Be aware of any factors affecting your client's food choice, e.g. therapeutic diet, religious beliefs, chewing difficulty, etc.
- Meal times can be made into an enjoyable social occasion. Try to ensure that the environment is conducive to eating and that food is attractively presented and served.
- As a carer you can help, support and encourage your client to eat a healthy diet, but ultimately you must respect your client's own choice of food and drink.

References

Department of Health (1991) *Dietary Reference Values for Food Energy and Nutrients for the United Kingdom.* (Report on Health and Social Subjects, 41.) HMSO, London.

Department of Health (1992) *The Nutrition of Elderly People.* (Report on Health and Social Subjects, 43.) HMSO, London.

Foodsense (1992) *The Food Safety Act 1990 and You. A Guide for the Food Industry.* HMSO Publication PBO 351. Available from Foodsense, London SE99 7TT (Tel: 081-694 8862).

Further reading

Burns, B. (1992) Working up a thirst. *Nursing Times,* 24 June, **88**(26), 44–5.

Greenhorn, T. (1992) Fed up. *Nursing Times,* 22 July, **88**(30), 32–3.

Girvin, J. (1991) Deals on meals, improving quality of patients' food. *Nursing Times,* 27 August, **87**(34), 38–40.

Health Education Authority (1990) *Guide to Healthy Eating.* Available from Health Promotion Departments.

Health Education Authority (1990) *From Milk to Mixed Feeding.* Available from Health Promotion Departments.

Holmes, S. (1991) Nutrition and surgical patients. *Nursing Standard,* **24**(44), 30–32.

Karmel, A. (1992) *The Complete Baby and Toddler Meal Planner.* Ebury Press, London.

Langley, J. (1988) *Working with Swallowing Disorders.* Winslow Press, Oxford.

Logemann, J. (1983) *Evaluation and Treatment of Swallowing Disorders.* College Hill Press, San Diego.

Mairis, E. (1992) An appetite life. Assessing and meeting nutritional needs. *Professional Nurse,* August, **7**(11), 732–7.

Ministry of Agriculture, Fisheries & Food (1991) *Food Additives.* Available free from Foodsense, London SE99 7TT (Tel: 081-694 8862).

Ministry of Agriculture, Fisheries & Food (1991) *Food Safety.* Available free from Foodsense, London SE99 7TT (Tel: 081-694 8862).

Peters, A. (1992) Half starved but not fed up. *Nursing,* 13 February, **5**(3), 4.

Robbins, C. (1985) *Eating for Health.* Granada Press.

Roper, N., Logan, T. & Tierney, A. (1980) *The Elements of Nursing,* Chapter 10. Churchill Livingstone, Edinburgh.

Williams, K. (1991) *Practical Approach to Caring,* Pitmans, London.

Chapter 10
Promoting Comfort, Rest, Sleep and Caring for the Client in Pain

Christine Cooper, Christine McMahon and Elizabeth Atchison

Overview

This chapter is in three sections. It covers the overall comfort of the patient and discusses how we can prevent pressure sores and the complications of immobility. Bed making, positioning the client and the use of aids to prevent pressure sores are included.

An explanation of the circadian rhythm and the stages of sleep is given, along with how we can promote sleep and adapt the environment and routine to facilitate sleep and rest.

Pain and its transmission are explored along with how to recognize when a client is in pain. The use of pain-killing drugs (analgesics) and the factors that affect the expression of pain are discussed. The final topic of discussion is how we, as carers, can help clients who are in discomfort or pain.

Key words

Immobile, pressure area/sore, decubitus ulcer, hyperaemic reaction, necrosis, shearing, contractures, deep vein thrombosis, exercise active/passive, position, circadian rhythm, stages of sleep, routines/behaviours, insomnia, environment, nursing intervention, acute/chronic pain, analgesic, pain threshold, pain pathway.

Pressure sores

I am sure that you have sat on a hard chair for a long time and been left feeling numb and sore. You will have consciously registered this discomfort and if the situation allowed it you would have wriggled in your seat or got up and walked about. The same also happens at night when you are asleep and during the night you change your position many times.

Activity 10.1 ■

 Can you list the reasons which could prevent a person changing their position when they become uncomfortable, providing they were aware of their discomfort.

■ ■

Your list may include:

■   Someone who is very weak and unable to move, especially if the bed clothes are restrictive;
■   A person who has undergone a stroke and lost the use of their arm or leg;
■   A person with a fractured leg who is on traction or in a plaster;
■   A deeply unconscious person will not be able to register the fact that they are uncomfortable and then change position.

In the case of a client who is unable to change position without assistance, their skin is subjected to pressure. Areas of skin particularly prone to this are those covering a bone which we sit or lie on. The supply of blood is reduced and after a period of time the tissues in the area will be affected by the deprivation of the oxygen and nutrients that the blood normally transports around the body to feed the cells in tissues. The cells die (*necrosis*) and a breakdown of the skin will result in a pressure sore (*decubitus ulcer*).

Factors which increase the risk of a pressure sore developing

Poor nutrition
A diet which is lacking in iron, vitamin C, protein and minerals such as zinc. These are needed to formulate haemaglobin in red blood cells to transport the oxygen to cells for energy and to keep skin generally healthy.

Cardiovascular system
This needs to be strong to circulate the blood around the body.

Incontinence
Whether of urine or faeces, incontinence increases the risk of pressure sores, therefore any incontinent client is a high risk.

Weight
The obese or very thin client is also at risk.

Mood
The mood of the client can also influence their risk of developing a pressure sore. Should the client be feeling despondent and fed up then they will be less motivated to move themselves about or take active steps to prevent pressure sores.

Immobility, tight clothing
It should be remembered that pressure sores can occur at any time should the client become *immobile*, whether or not they are in bed. Tight clothing, especially jeans or buttons on seat pockets, can cause pressure leading to a pressure sore.

Visual indicators of pressure sore development

Activity 10.2   ■

 Place one arm on a table and then lean your other elbow on it and press down. How does it feel? Keep on pressing. What can you see when you finally remove your elbow?

■ ■

At first you will feel pain and discomfort and you would normally remove your elbow and stop the pain. In order to feel pain you need nerves to take the *pain message* to the brain and you need to be conscious to receive and interpret the message. Then you need functioning muscles to remove your elbow to prevent any damage to the tissues.

Keep on pressing and you will see the result of direct pressure on the skin where it is covering a bone. When you eventually remove your arm look at the area that was directly under your elbow. At first this area will be paler and feel cool due to the lack of blood supply, then it will very quickly change colour – to look darker and red. Place the back of a bent finger over the area and you should feel heat. This is the effect of the body acknowledging the fact that the specific area has been starved of blood and that it needs oxygen to feed the tissues – hence the increased blood supply. This is called a hyperaemic reaction.

Do not rub the area as this will only interrupt what nature is trying to do to overcome the effect of prolonged pressure. It has been shown that rubbing an area can actually cause damage to the small blood vessels (capillaries) in the skin. This is also a predisposing factor for the development of a pressure sore.

Look again in about 15 minutes to see if the redness and heat have disappeared. The length of time the redness stays is dictated by the length of time the pressure was applied. Should a hyperaemic reaction last longer than an hour then there is a possibility of tissue damage.

When changing the position of a client, look at the pressure areas for any signs of redness and heat. If such signs are present, report them to the registered practitioner, as it could be an indication that the client needs their position changing more frequently.

Tissue damage and pressure sore development

Activity 10.3   ■

 Place your lower arm on a table with the elbow at the edge. Pressing down hard on your arm pull your elbow towards you and over the end of the table.

You will note that your skin has stayed in the same place whilst your bones (radius and ulnar) have moved.

■ ■

The same effect happens when a client slides down from a sitting position in bed – their skin stays in the same position whilst their sacral bone slides down. This effect is called *shearing* and is thought to be the cause of pressure sores developing under the skin and then breaking the surface. It is caused by stretching and damage to the capillaries in the skin and by the subsequent interruption of the blood supply to the tissues.

Incorrect lifting techniques, resulting in clients being dragged up the bed, will cause both friction and shearing, leading to tissue damage and a pressure sore.

Therefore careful attention should be paid to handling, lifting and positioning clients to prevent the development of pressure sores. Refer to the chapter on client handling.

Areas prone to pressure (Fig. 10.1)

Activity 10.4   ■

I presume that you will have been sitting in more or less the same position for the last half an hour or so whilst you have been reading. Can you list the parts of you that feel discomfort?

They could include:

- Buttocks, sacral area
- Backs of your legs, especially if the chair is the wrong size for you

Now lie down on a hard floor flat on your back without a pillow, if you can bear it. Try and stay there for about five minutes. Consider which parts of your body are feeling uncomfortable.

Your list could include:

- Buttocks (sacral area)
- Heels
- Shoulder blades (scapulae)
- Spine (vertebrae)
- Head (occipital)

Now turn over and lie on your side. What parts of the body do you find uncomfortable now?

You may include:

- Hip (ischial tuberosity, pelvis)
- Shoulder, upper arm
- Ankle
- Ear
- Sides of your knees

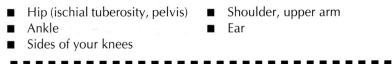

Comparing your lists you will see that the sacral area (buttocks) is mentioned twice; this is in fact the most common place for a pressure sore to occur.

Fig. 10.1 Areas prone to
pressure.

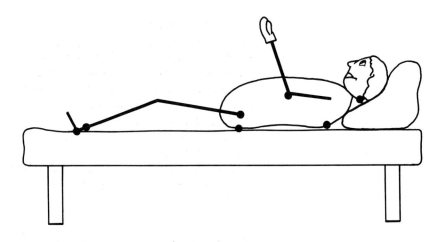

Measures to prevent pressure sores

Prevention is better than cure: Should a pressure sore occur then it can
take weeks or months to heal, resulting in extreme discomfort and pain for
the client. Much has been written on the causes and prevention of pressure
sores and within this chapter we can only explain the principles. I would
recommend you to refer to the Further Reading section at the end of this
chapter.

The client's *care plan* will indicate the actions to be taken to prevent
pressure sores. These may include:

- Regular changing of the client's position, maybe every two hours. It
  may be advantageous to use a *turning chart* to record and plan
  whether the client is on their right or left side or whether they are
  sitting up. The position of the client can be predetermined to ensure
  that they are in a suitable position for meal times, i.e. sitting up to
  facilitate eating.
- Keeping the skin clean and dry, especially if the client is incontinent or
  pyrexial and perspiring a great deal.
- The use of special mattresses and pillows which relieve pressure in
  vulnerable areas.
- Application of special dressings in areas where the skin is sore and
  liable to breakdown (usually the sacrum and hip).

When attending to hygiene needs the carer must always observe the skin
for the *early signs* of the effect of pressure and immediately report any
signs of redness or skin abrasions.

Positioning the client

Should you be in an uncomfortable position then, as we have already
discussed, you will wriggle around to get comfortable. There are times

Fig. 10.2 Assisting a client to change position by sitting him forward.

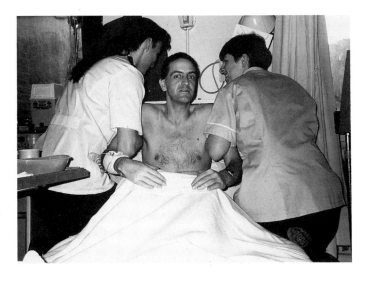

when we as carers will have to position a client when they are unable to do this for themselves (Fig. 10.2).

Should the client have any damage to their nervous system following a stroke or spinal injury, be unconscious or be frail and weak then they will be at risk of developing stiffness of joints which could develop into contractures. This occurs in the hip, knee and elbow joints, resulting in the client lying on their side in a fetal position (curled up with their knees bent towards their chest). Clients with rheumatoid arthritis may also need special attention to their position and a splint applied to their wrist, for example.

After assessment by a registered practitioner a plan of care will be drawn up. By referring to this we can then position the client using soft pillows and any appropriate aids. Care must be taken to ensure no excess pressure is exerted on the shoulder when the client is on their side in bed. The lower arm and shoulder should be gently eased into position after the client has been turned on to their side.

Feet and wrists need to be well supported to avoid drop foot or wrist; excess pressure on the calf muscles must be avoided to prevent a *deep vein thrombosis* (DVT). A thrombosis is a clot in the veins. The constant movement of our feet and ankles usually helps to pump the blood back up to the heart. Sometimes lack of exercise and pressure on the lower limbs in conjunction with dehydration will inhibit the flow of blood, resulting in the formation of a clot. There is a danger of the clot moving up from the leg and lodging in a blood vessel in the lungs, causing a pulmonary embolus and endangering the client's life.

Exercise

Passive and if possible active exercise will help to overcome some of the problems mentioned in the previous section and the physiotherapist plays a major role in this aspect of care.

Activity 10.5 ■■■■■■■■■■■■■■■■■■■■■■■■■■■

 While sitting in a chair, raise your left leg and, placing your right hand under your calf, rotate your foot and move it up and down. Can you feel the muscles contracting?

■■■■■■■■■■■■■■■■■■■■■■■■■■■■■■■■■■

This movement helps to return the blood to the heart and normally occurs when we walk. Immobile clients should therefore undertake some form of foot or ankle exercise at regular intervals.

Further complications of immobility

The immobile client may suffer from many more complications. Some examples are:

- Constipation – due to the lack of exercise and stimulus, and perhaps also to a change in diet.
- Anorexia – or a general lack of interest in eating and drinking (refer to Chapter 9 for more detailed coverage of nutrition).
- Calcium moving from the bone – this can occur on long-term bed rest and can lead to kidney stones (renal calculi). It may occur in the client with a spinal injury. The removal of the calcium from the bones to the blood stream will have a weakening effect on the bone (osteoporosis). This could result in bone fracture – usually the neck of the femur – and can occur when the client gets out of bed for the first time after a long period of inactivity.
- Depression and frustration – may affect the client due to the change in dependency and life style, resulting in various mood changes. Plans of care should include ways to maintain the client's interest in the family, friends and hobbies. The occupational therapist can help the client in various forms of diversional therapeutic activities, which may be designed to maintain physical co-ordination and alignment. Some areas of work have activities organizers, who help to create a stimulating and pleasant environment.

Activity 10.6 ■■■■■■■■■■■■■■■■■■■■■■■■■■

 Consider how you can maintain interests, family and friend contacts with your clients.

■■■■■■■■■■■■■■■■■■■■■■■■■■■■■■■■■■

Your list may include:

- Free access for family and friends
- Portable telephone with money or card available
- Facilities to read out and reply to letters
- Mobile library visiting the client
- Radio and television, at the client's request
- Jigsaws, cards and games
- Knitting, marquetry

This section only covers this topic briefly and you should ask around in your own organization to find out what is available for clients.

Bed making

A comfortable bed is extremely important for the client and individual needs in terms of number of pillows and blankets must be considered.

Health and safety

Refer to Chapter 5 on mobility and safer client handling.

- Always remember that if a bed has brakes, they must be on.
- If the bed can be raised, bring it up to a safe working height. If the client is in their own home it may be necessary to kneel down to keep your back straight.
- If fire blankets are in use, check these are correctly positioned and attached.

Cross-infection

- Hands must be washed between each client and plastic aprons should be worn by the carer (refer to Chapter 6 concerning the control of infection).
- Assess what clean linen is required and only take what is necessary to prevent contamination of clean linen. A linen skip should be close at hand and any linen contaminated with body fluids must be put into the correctly coloured bag (Fig. 10.3).
- Bed clothes should be removed with care to prevent air currents and micro-organisms travelling from one client to another. The bed clothes should be folded neatly on to two chairs or the rack/shelf on the bed, taking care to keep them off the floor.
- Any equipment such as pillows or bed cradles must be placed on a chair near to the client – never on the floor or on someone else's bed.

Principles of bed making

- Ensure a smooth bottom sheet with no wrinkles or crumbs.
- Bed clothes should be loose enough to allow movement, i.e. sheets and blankets should have a tuck put into them to prevent pressure on toes, heels or ankles. (Duvets are lighter and allow more movement.)

Fig. 10.3 Disposal of
soiled linen.

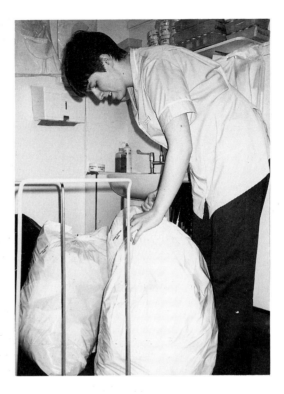

- Pillows should be positioned to give support to the back if the client is sitting up.
- Careful explanation should be given to the client and their co-operation sought if possible.
- Should the client be in the bed, then changing bed linen and remaking the bed is often performed at the same time as meeting hygiene needs. The clean bottom sheet can be inserted with the client on their side after they have had their back washed. All this needs careful preparation and the sheet should be rolled up before the client is washed. It is a procedure that is best undertaken with two people in order to support and help to turn the client.
- If the client is lying on a special mattress, such as a low air loss bed or ripple mattress connected to an electric pump, or one that is filled with siliconized hollow fibres, care must be taken in tucking in the bottom sheet as this could interfere with the function of the mattress. Always refer to the manufacturer's instructions; in fact many firms will come and demonstrate the correct use of their equipment.

Sleep

Sleep is important to us all and the average person spends about one-third of their lives asleep. This section gives an explanation of our normal sleep cycle and how we can assist a patient to sleep and rest.

Circadian rhythm

Our daily lives are influenced by our *circadian rhythm*, which is a daily cycle and our biological clock. A number of factors influence this clock, such as light and dark, and various social cues such as increased traffic noise first thing in the morning. These act as reminders as to the time of the day.

During the *day* we are actively moving about, eating and using energy. Our body prepares for this by producing a hormone (adrenaline) that helps to keep us awake and alert; this is very much influenced by light. Our blood pressure and pulse rise during the day, reaching their maximum between 12.00 and 18.00 hours, whilst our temperature is at its maximum between 18.00 and 24.00 hours.

During the *evening* our adrenaline levels fall and we begin to find it more difficult to concentrate as our body is preparing for sleep both mentally and physically.

During the *night* the body and mind rest and sleep, with the blood pressure, pulse and temperature being lowest between 02.00 and 06.00 hours. It is during this time of inactivity that growth and repair of tissues such as skin, bone and bone marrow are thought to take place (Closs, 1988).

Early morning, from about 04.00 hours, the body is preparing for activity and adrenaline is produced.

Should our normal routine and sleep patterns change, this will have an effect on us. For instance, jet lag occurs when we travel across time zones and our normal circadian rhythm (sleep/wake cycle) is altered. This is experienced in particular when we travel from West to East because we experience sunset earlier than our body expects and we are trying to persuade our body clock that it is time to go to sleep earlier than usual.

Importance of sleep

Sleep is something we all need and there are many theories about why we need it.

Activity 10.7 ■

 Make a list of the reasons why you feel sleep is important.

■ ■

Your list may include:

■ The brain needs time for a rest in order to sweep away unnecessary memories and consolidate learning
■ The body needs time to rest and sleep has a restorative function
■ Sleep aids the process of healing wounds
■ It makes us 'healthy and wise'

You may find it easier to identify what happens to us if we do not get enough sleep (i.e. sleep deprivation).

Activity 10.8   ■

 Make a list of the effects of sleep deprivation.

■ ■

Your list may include:

- Not being able to concentrate
- Being lethargic
- Being antisocial
- Feeling tired, which could lead to chronic fatigue
- Being irritable
- Increase in stress levels
- Becoming depressed

I am sure that you have felt these effects yourself to some degree and you will certainly have seen them in clients.

Time spent in sleep

We spend up to a third of our lives asleep and the length of our sleep periods changes throughout our lives (Fig. 10.4). This is of course individual and can be dependent on culture and habits. Many prime ministers in the past have managed on very little sleep, less than four hours a night, whilst others had a longer sleep plus a nap in the afternoon.

There are two types of sleep: non-REM (no rapid eye movement) and REM (rapid eye movement). *Non-REM sleep* has four different stages, 1 to 4, as described below. The sleeper passes through these four stages in cycles, going from light to deep sleep and then the sequence reverses, going from deep to light sleep. *REM sleep* comes at the end of each sleep cycle and is a much lighter sleep, during which the eyes move rapidly from side to side below closed eyelids. It is during this stage that dreams occur. The client moves about and changes position and any snoring will cease.

Fig. 10.4 Time spent in bed.

Baby
16 hours out of 24 hours

Teenager
10–11 hours a night

Adult
7 hours a night

Elderly
5–7 hours a night plus naps during the day

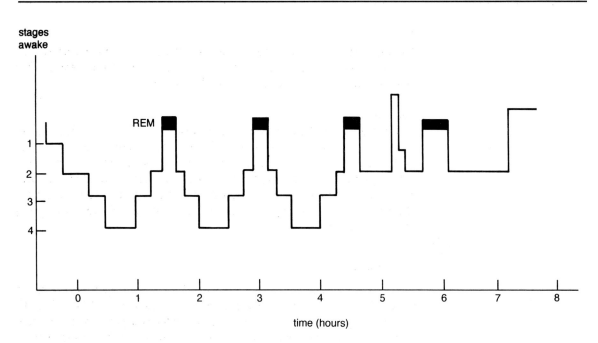

Fig. 10.5 Sleep cycle. (Adapted from Gribbon, 1990.)

The sleep cycle

A complete sleep cycle lasts about 90 minutes and is repeated about four or five times during an average eight hour night's sleep. Therefore a full cycle could be stages 1 to 4, then 4 to 1 with REM sleep between each cycle (Fig. 10.5). As the client falls asleep the brain becomes less responsive to outside stimuli and the body relaxes.

Non-REM sleep

Stage 1
This is when the client falls asleep. The body begins to relax and all the vital signs (temperature, pulse, respiration and blood pressure) are normal. The client can be easily awoken at this time. This stage lasts about 20 minutes. If it lasts more than 40 minutes then the client is thought to be suffering from insomnia.

Stage 2
This is a period of light sleep, when brain activity begins to slow down.

Stage 3
The muscles become relaxed and the vital signs become depressed as sleep becomes heavier.

Stage 4
During this stage of deep sleep, arousal is difficult; the vital signs are at their lowest. However the digestive tract is very active during this stage. This stage of deep sleep is reduced in the elderly client.

REM sleep
This is a much lighter sleep and can last from 5 to 15 minutes. It occurs at the end of each cycle between each Stage 1 sleep. The blood flow to the brain increases and the patient dreams and moves about more. This stage is thought to be necessary to keep us sane, and although we do not always remember our dreams, we all do dream and you may well be aware of them should you awake during this stage. We tend to consolidate our learning during this stage.

?

Did you know?

Problem solving can be incorporated in a dream. A group of nine students were asked to identify the next two letters in a sequence of O T T F F. The next day it was found that two students solved the problem before they went to bed and the other seven solved it in a dream. (The answer is S S; they are the first letters of the numbers one to seven) (Gribbon, 1990).

Factors that influence sleep.

Activity 10.9 ■

Can you list anything that could induce sleep?

■ ■

Your list could include:

- Having a hot milky drink
- Reading
- Having a warm bath to relax

- Keeping to a certain routine
- Listening to music

Admission to hospital and changes to life style may alter sleep patterns.

Change in routine
Routines change when people enter some sort of communal life and it can be difficult to meet everyone's individual needs. During our life we become *conditioned* in our preparation to go to sleep, our brain learns this from an early age. For instance, keeping to the same routine for a child is important to induce sleep and should the normal bedtime story be missed, the child may find it difficult to get off to sleep.

Keeping to a routine of specific behaviour informs the brain that we are getting ready for bed and these messages are relayed to other parts of the brain and body, inducing sleep.

Activity 10.10 ■■■■■■■■■■■■■■■■■■■■■■■■■■■■

 Consider your normal routine before going to bed and sleep.

■■■■■■■■■■■■■■■■■■■■■■■■■■■■■■■■■■

It may include:

- Taking the dog out for a walk
- Locking up the house
- Having a drink of hot chocolate
- Having a bath and putting on your night clothes
- Brushing your teeth
- Reading in bed or listening to the radio
- Turning off lights

It is important to find out how long a client normally sleeps, what time they go to bed and what routine they follow before going to sleep. Adapting their care to comply with their normal routine as much as possible will not only make the patient feel more secure in the environment, but will help them to get off to sleep. This will help overcome *initial insomnia* which occurs at sleep onset; *racing mind phenomena* or anxiety will make this type of insomnia worse.

Milky drinks can help promote sleep, as we see in advertisements for Bournvita and Horlicks.

A substance called tryptophan, which is found in milk, beef and beans, is thought to promote sleep onset; whilst 500 mg caffeine, equivalent to three cups of coffee drunk over 24 hours, can disrupt sleep.

Sleep can be reduced by 20 to 25% when a patient goes into hospital. I am sure that you have experienced a patient complaining of lack of sleep whilst in hospital, and looking forward to going home for a good night's sleep!

Activity 10.11 ■■■■■■■■■■■■■■■■■■■■■■■■■■■

 List anything that could prevent someone getting off to sleep.

■■■■■■■■■■■■■■■■■■■■■■■■■■■■■■■■■

Your list could include:

- Noise from people talking and moving about, and from equipment
- Pain and discomfort
- Anxiety
- Bladder distension
- Difficulty in breathing
- Change in surroundings
- Unfamiliar noises and lights, and the close proximity of other people
- Room too hot and stuffy or too cold

- Being either linked to monitoring equipment or in close proximity to someone who is

How can we help promote sleep?

Reduce pain and promote comfort

This topic is considered in more depth in the section concerning pain. The main principles we should consider are described here.

- Sometimes by changing position and using a supportive mattress and pillows, a client can be made more comfortable.
- Massage can relax a client and, used in conjunction with aromatherapy, can reduce anxiety and induce sleep.
- Analgesics should be administered to control pain, and maintenance doses should be given before the client complains of severe pain. It is important to monitor and evaluate the level of pain and the effect of analgesics.
- A full bladder will prevent restful sleep. Always ensure a client has had the opportunity to pass urine before settling down to sleep and be prepared for the client waking in the night to pass urine. It is essential for a patient to have a means of attracting a carer's attention during the night. For the ambulant client positioning of the bed near to a toilet or a commode will reduce the incidence of falls.

Reduce anxiety and stress

Anyone in a new environment will be anxious due to concern over their illness or to separation from their family, friends or a pet. This anxiety stimulates the body and prevents sleep. We all need information and *fear of the unknown* is an obvious cause of stress. The following may help reduce anxiety and stress:

- Spending time listening to and talking with a client is very supportive and can help someone to settle down to sleep (Fig. 10.6). Clients with sleeping problems need to be shown both empathy and understanding.
- Relaxation by listening to music or reading may help to induce sleep; however for some patients these may act as stimuli and raise the arousal level and inhibit the onset of sleep.
- Allowing visitors or pets to stay with a client as they settle down to sleep may be beneficial. Providing a patient with access to a telephone so they can chat to their family is also very helpful.

Aid breathing and help to prevent gastro-oesophageal reflux (indigestion)

If a client is helped into a more upright position this may facilitate breathing and help control reflux (when the contents of the stomach pass up into the oesophagus).

Fig. 10.6 Listening and
talking to a client.

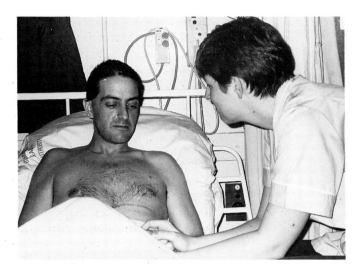

Reduce noise level

We are not always aware of the level of noise around a client.

Activity 10.12 ■

Consider what increases the noise level in your care environment during
the night.

■ ■

You could have included any of the following:

- Squeaky equipment, trolleys, shoes, doors
- Other clients
- Client call systems, telephones, conversation, radio and television
- Confused and ill clients requiring care
- Admissions during the night
- External noises such as traffic, aeroplanes

Some of these causes may be out of our control, but if we prepare the
client by explaining the cause of the noise, it may help them to accept it
and so cope better. We should be aware that although we need stimuli to
keep us awake and alert during the night the client does not, so we must
make every effort to reduce the noise level in the care area.

As we grow older we become more sensitive to noise. Consider how a
young baby, once they are off to sleep, can sleep through door bells
ringing, radio and television; an older person, however, quickly wakes up if
they hear an unfamiliar sound. We need to consider this fact when caring
for the elderly and ensure the care environment is quiet and conducive to
sleep. It was found that noise was the main reason for clients taking
sleeping tablets whilst in hospital (Closs, 1988).

Light

This is a stimulant and it acts on our brain and tells us that we should be awake and alert. It also makes the body produce hormones that enable us to be active (think of the sun waking you up in the morning).

It may be beneficial for a client to have some sort of night light on, or a light switch nearby, as it enables them to orientate themselves to a new environment or ensures that they can find their way around a familiar one and avoid falls.

Temperature of the environment

This needs to be warm but not stuffy; an ideal temperature is about 20°C. There also needs to be an adequate amount of fresh air to promote sleep. As we grow older our temperature control mechanism tends to diminish. As our body temperature drops during sleep it is important to maintain a constant ambient temperature of 21°C for the elderly and ensure they have light but warm night clothes and bed clothes.

Nursing interventions

The more critically ill or dependent a client is, the more they are disturbed during the night and are unable to complete a normal sleep cycle. This can lead to sleep deprivation, resulting in possible confusion and, in the case of a surgical client, a delay in wound healing.

Care needs to be planned with as little disturbance as possible. Aim to give only essential care to a client during the night, so they may complete a full sleep cycle.

Pain

The purpose of this section is to explore the concept of pain. Caring for clients in pain can be extremely demanding, especially emotionally.

It is important to state from the beginning that pain is an individual unique experience. We can never make assumptions about a client's pain. For example, if two clients have the same operation they may not experience the same amount of pain. It is often easy to say 'Mr Smith is up and around now but Mr Bloggs is not, he must be making a fuss'.

A client's pain is 'whatever the patient says it is and exists whenever he says it does' (McCaffery, 1983).

What is pain?

Activity 10.13 ■

 What is pain? This may seem like a simple question. Spend some time writing down your thoughts.

■ ■

You may have noted some of the following:

- The body's way of telling you there is something wrong
- Warning sign
- Sign to show you are getting worse
- Response to injury
- Unpleasant feeling/ experience
- Sign to show you are healing
- Sensation to stop you doing further harm

You may have had many more, all of which may be correct because pain means different things to different people. We know of times when people experience pain without a physical cause; this does not mean their pain is not real. Likewise we know of people who have walked miles from an accident on a broken leg to get help, yet felt no pain at the time!

I hope you are able to see just how complex the concept of pain is. In an attempt to unravel it let's start by looking at how the pain message reaches the brain.

The pain message

Activity 10.14 ■

When you last stubbed your toe or trapped your finger what did you do?

■ ■

In your answer you may have to include:

- Rubbed it
- Screamed
- Repeated certain words
- Jumped up and down
- Shouted

or perhaps nothing until a time which was more convenient.

We have nerves or fibres all over the body which, when injury occurs, start to send a message. This message travels along the nerve and we often refer to this as a pathway. The message continues along the pathway to the spinal cord and then up to the brain. At the point where the message enters the spinal cord is an area we call the *gate*. This gate may be closed, stopping the pain message travelling up the spinal cord, and hence the brain does not receive the message of pain. Or the gate may be open, allowing the pain message to travel up the spinal cord, thus reaching the brain. The brain then tells us we are in pain and we react or behave in a way which may be the same as other people or individual to us.

Along the same pathway that the pain message uses also travel other messages like *touch*, i.e. rubbing. If there are two message trying to use the same pathway at the same time, i.e. pain *and* touch, only so much of either message can get it through. This explains why rubbing an area lessens the pain temporarily (Figs. 10.7 and 10.8).

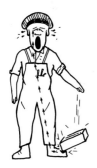

Fig. 10.7 Worker dropping a brick on his foot.

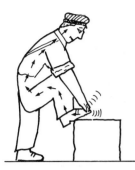

Fig. 10.8 Worker rubbing affected foot.

There is one further important fact to consider. Our brain interprets the pain message. Our brain is also capable of stopping the pain message. We do this in two ways. We may ignore the message, which allows us to act normally – for example walking on a broken leg to get help. Alternatively we may send a second message back down the spinal cord that blocks our original pain message. It is thought that hypnosis and relaxation work in this way. This also demonstrates the importance of our state of mind in controlling and tolerating pain (Fig. 10.9). However, this is only part of the picture and it is not just a case of 'mind over matter'. We will look at this again later on.

How do we know a patient is in pain?

Activity 10.15 ■

 Make a list of the ways you would know a client was in pain if they were unable to tell you.

■ ■

You may have recorded the following suggestions:

■ Facial expression   ■ Clammy
■ Hunched up   ■ Pale
■ Rubbing   ■ Reduced appetite
■ Crying   ■ Being sick
■ Moaning   ■ Being quiet
■ Sweating   ■ Raised pulse

It is important to remember that if the pain has gone on for a long time many of the above signs may not be present. Clients who have had long term pain may appear on the surface to be pain free. Do not assume this to be the case.

In a study looking at pain, 68% of nurses thought the client would tell them if they had pain and needed a pain killer. However, 42% of clients expected and assumed the nurses would know! (Hayward, 1975; Seers, 1987).

Fig. 10.9 Worker carrying on despite initial pain.

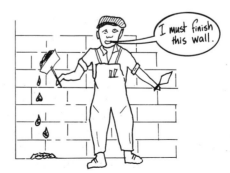

'Everyone knows what their own pain is like, but no one knows what anybody else's pain feels like' (Fry, 1977). Asking is the first step to understanding.

Factors which affect the way individuals respond to pain

All of the following must be considered when caring for the client in pain (Seers, 1988).

Family influence
Adult responses to pain may well have been shaped by childhood. For example if a hurt child cries it may be cuddled, or alternatively it may be ignored and praised when it stops crying.

Social influence
The response of others to our complaints of pain may affect the way we behave.

Cultural influences
There has been much research into the influences of culture on a person's responses to pain. It appears some people from some cultures prefer to be alone when in pain and others prefer company. Perhaps more importantly, some cultures do not express their pain through words (*stiff upper lip*) while others are used to expressing their pain more loudly.

It is important to remember that none of the examples above mean an individual is either making a fuss or has no pain.

The meaning of pain
Some people may view pain as a punishment; others may see pain as a necessary part of life, which will be relieved in an after life.

Language
A language barrier can prevent patients from verbally expressing their pain. Being unable to express pain may result in fear and uncertainty. It is particularly important to ask a client about pain, through either the family or an interpreter.

Part of the body
Some body areas are more easy to discuss than others!

Acute and chronic pain

Now we have looked at how we experience pain, we can begin to look at two broad categories of pain: acute and chronic.

Acute pain
Acute pain is defined by several things:

- It persists for a short length of time.
- It often gets better quickly.
- It is often associated with healing, for example following surgery.

Chronic pain
Chronic pain is associated with different things:

- It usually gets worse
- It is often associated with a deteriorating problem
- It has a constant/long time span

Activity 10.16 ■

Make two lists, one called *chronic pain* and one called *acute pain*. In each list note down some of the causes of each type of pain.

■ ■

Here are some examples:

Acute pain
- Sudden injury
- Appendicitis
- Headache
- Toothache

Chronic pain
- Backache
- Arthritis
- Cancer pain

Sometimes an acute pain can become chronic if it persists and the underlying cause is not treated.

Pain-killing drugs (analgesics)

The reason for giving pain-killing drugs is different for the two categories of pain. For *acute pain* our aim is to give pain-killing drugs for a short time and then to reduce and stop them quickly as the pain improves. For *chronic pain* we often give strong analgesics such as morphine. Often the dose needs to be increased regularly. We also give these analgesics to keep the pain away and the client pain free. It is therefore not unusual to be still giving the analgesic when the client has no pain. In fact we would wish to keep our client completely free of pain.

There are many different analgesics we can use to control all types of pain and the doctor and nurse will usually decide. For clients in pain we usually follow the guidelines shown in Fig. 10.10 and move up the rungs of the ladder until we reach a drug that works.

Routes of administration
Analgesic drugs can be given in several ways:

- In tablet form (orally), depending on the drugs, either four hourly or, if in a slow release form, 12 hourly.

Fig. 10.10 Analgesics work by blocking the pain message. (World Health Organization, 1986).

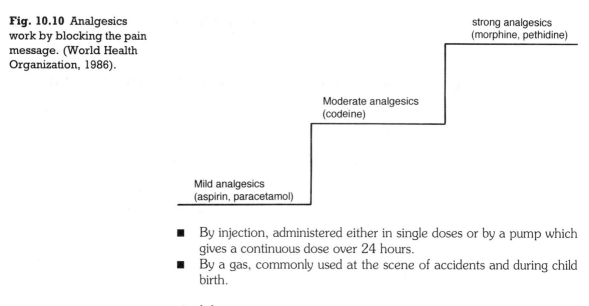

- By injection, administered either in single doses or by a pump which gives a continuous dose over 24 hours.
- By a gas, commonly used at the scene of accidents and during child birth.

Activity 10.17 ■

 In view of what you know now what alternative methods might we use to control pain *other* than medicines?

■ ■

You may have thought of the following:

- Gentle rubbing or massage (not bony areas or pressure areas, check with the person in charge first): *touch*
- Changing position: *physical comfort*
- Making client comfortable: *physical comfort*
- Talking to them: *mental comfort*
- Relaxation: *mental comfort*
- Diversion, e.g. music, art: *mental comfort*
- Just being with them: *mental comfort*

There are some other methods which come under the heading of complementary therapies, such as aromatherapy, hypnosis, reflexology and acupuncture. Whilst these are not yet seen widely in hospitals, their use has been given much more consideration recently.

Pain threshold

The pain threshold is the limit to which an individual can tolerate pain before it becomes unacceptable. The pain threshold is unique to the individual. The pain threshold may alter in the same individual and is greatly influenced by the state of mind. It is therefore something we can help to increase and hence ease distress.

Activity 10.18   ■

What factors do you think would raise or lower an individual's tolerance of pain?

■ ■

Under *raising the pain threshold* (higher tolerance of pain) you may have included:

- Being relaxed
- Low stress
- Being kept informed
- Loved
- Not alone

- Happy
- Low anxiety
- Comfortable
- Supported

Under *lowering the pain threshold* (lower tolerance to pain) you may have included:

- Fear
- Stress
- Unsure of what is happening
- Sad

- Anxiety
- Lack of sleep
- Alone
- Expectation of severe pain

The role of the carer in pain control

We have covered a great deal of ground on the topic of pain. It is now time to summarize this and examine the carer's role.

Clients may experience *acute* or *chronic* pain. In both cases, the patient can expect to become pain free. It may sometimes take a short time to find the appropriate analgesic and dose.

It is important as carers to report to the nurse in charge or doctor if a particular drug is not working. It is usual that most drugs will take effect within half an hour of their administration. Speedy reporting allows the client to become pain free quicker and alerts staff to the fact that a drug is no longer working. We also discussed how we might see if a client was in pain but unable to tell us. This again needs observing and reporting.

As carers, we may offer many of the comforting actions discussed under the section on *alternative methods of pain control*, such as *touch* (if agreed by the nurse in charge), *relaxation* and *positioning*.

In the section on the *pain threshold* we discussed how we might raise clients' tolerance to pain and ease their distress. Again many of these actions can be performed by the carer, for example *reassurance*, *company* if required and *support*. If necessary, find a nurse or doctor to answer patients' questions and worries.

Finally it is most important never to judge a client but to continue with an individual approach to care. The client knows their own pain best but we can share in supporting them at this difficult time. Good communication and understanding are the key.

Summary

In this chapter we have considered the rest, comfort and pain control of the patient. The causes and prevention of pressure sores were explained and advice given on how to maintain the comfort of a client confined to bed or with limited mobility. We hope that it has given you an insight into the importance of maintaining movement and the prevention of pressure sores, not only considering the physical aspects of care but also the psychological ones.

The final section considered the pain pathway and the other messages that use the same pathway such as touch. Finally we considered the state of mind of the patient and the role of the carer.

References

Closs, J. (1988) Patients' sleep–wake rhythms in hospital. Part one. *Nursing Times*, 6 January, **84**(1), 48–50.

Closs, J. (1988) Patients' sleep-wake rhythms in hospital. Part two. *Nursing Times*, 13 January, **84**(2), 54–5.

Fry, E. (1977) Post operative analgesia. *Nursing Times*, 2 December, **83**(84), 37–8.

Gribbon, M. (1990) All in a night's sleep. *New Scientist*, 7 July, No. 1724, 1–4.

Haywood, J. (1975) *Information – a prescription against pain*. Royal College of Nursing, London.

Kearnes, S. (1989) Insomnia in the elderly. *Nursing Times*, 22 November, **85**(47), 32–3.

McCaffery, M. (1983) *Nursing the Patient in Pain*. Harper and Row, London.

Seers, K. (1987) Perceptions of pain. *Nursing Times*, **83**(48), 37–8.

Seers, K. (1988) Factors affecting pain assessment. *Professional Nurse*, **3**(6), 203–4.

World Health Organization (1986) *Cancer Pain Relief*. WHO, Geneva.

Further reading

Boomer, H. (1991) Getting children to sleep. *Nursing Times*, 20 March, **88**(48), 40–43.

Dias, B. (1992) Things that go bump in the night. *Nursing Times*, 16 September, **88**(38), 36–38.

East, E. (1992) How much does it hurt? *Nursing Times*, 30 September, **88**(40), 48–9.

Hill, L. (1992) The question of pressure. *Nursing Times*, 18 March, **88**(12), 76–82.

Malone, C. (1992) Intensive pressure. *Nursing Times*, 2 September, **88**(36), 57–62.

McCaffery, M. (1983) *Nursing the Patient in Pain*. Harper and Row, London.

Sofaer, B. (1984) *Pain; a Handbook for Nurses*. Harper and Row, London.

Walker, J. (1992) Living with pain. *Nursing Times*, 23 October, **88**(43), 28–32.

Willis, J. (1989) A good night's sleep. *Nursing Times*, 22 November, **85**(47), 29–31.

Section 3
Endorsements for Care in Specific Situations

Chapter 11
Clinical Investigations and Treatments
Jenny Partridge

Overview

In this chapter we explore ways in which carers can ease the fears and anxieties felt by clients as they face the prospect of investigations and treatments.

Key words

Information, reassurance, preparation, procedures.

Answering clients' questions

Whilst carers work within a familiar environment, clients may find these surroundings strange and unfamiliar and they are often anxious and hesitant in asking questions about what may be happening to them.

Activity 11.1 ■

Think back to when you started in your role or, if you can't remember, think of a time when you were working outside your usual workplace. How did you feel? Who did you go to for reassurance? Who answered your questions?

■ ■

You may have been in the very happy position of not feeling that you needed any *reassurance* as people answered your questions as you asked them or, even better, anticipated your needs and explained routines and rationales before you had a need to ask. However, it is more likely that you wandered around feeling, if not looking, a little lost and confused, wondering who to ask and whether they would think your question silly. Indeed, should you really know the answer!

Overall it is the responsibility of the qualified staff to ensure that individual clients receive the correct *information* about any investigation or treatment that will be undertaken. It is also likely that the client will question you as the person near them physically and someone who often appears more approachable, to gain clarification and possible further interpretation of the explanation they have already received.

All *procedures* carried out for the client by staff may be perceived as a clinical examination and therefore lead to great *anxiety*. This anxiety may not be overtly expressed but must never be ignored and should be anticipated by carers.

Activity 11.2 ■■■■■■■■■■■■■■■■■■■■■■■■■

List as many treatments and investigations as you can which are carried out for clients in your work area.

■■■■■■■■■■■■■■■■■■■■■■■■■■■■■■

The area that you work in and clients whom you care for will govern the range of treatments and investigations which you have identified. One example may be taking blood from a client (Fig. 11.1).

Activity 11.3 ■■■■■■■■■■■■■■■■■■■■■■■■■

Can you briefly explain what each of the investigations and treatments you have written down in Activity 11.2 means to the patient?

■■■■■■■■■■■■■■■■■■■■■■■■■■■■■■

Having a brief idea of what is required of each investigation and treatment will assist you in part of your role of *preparation*, *support* and *recovery* of the client and equipment.

Activity 11.4 ■■■■■■■■■■■■■■■■■■■■■■■■■

What does the client need to know about the treatment or investigation?

■■■■■■■■■■■■■■■■■■■■■■■■■■■■■■

Fig. 11.1 Obtaining a blood sample.

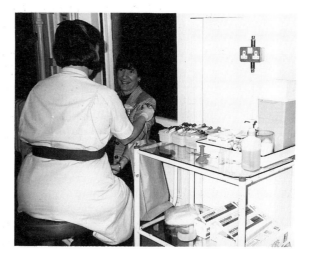

Clients' responses to information given may vary, but a clue may be had in these six words as identified by Rudyard Kipling in 'The Elephant's Child' one of the *Just So* stories. They are:

What? Why? When? How? Where? and Who?

It is likely that your client's questions will cover most of these, even though they may not express them as such. It is well known that *fear of the unknown* leads to a high degree of apprehension which affects the client (Boore, 1978; Hayward, 1975).

Of course it is likely that within your role you will be unable to answer all the questions, but at least you can refer to the qualified staff and raise awareness of the client's anxieties. Giving the client accurate *information* gives them *reassurance* and increases their understanding and control of the situation.

Preparation of the client

Any treatment or investigation is likely to start with some type of *preparation*. It may be in the form of preparing the client themselves, or the next of kin, depending on the client, the environment or the equipment.

It may be your role to assist in the preparation or to undertake some of the preparation on your own, so you will need to be aware of the instructions relating to equipment you may handle and the safe working practices that need to be adopted.

Anyone undergoing a procedure, be it investigation or treatment, will have given their consent. Consent may be written or verbal, assumed or asked (Fig. 11.2). This consent may be given by the client themselves or, if they are under the age of 16, by their parent/guardian. The judgement of whether the individual is able to give consent lies with the medical and nursing staff and there are guidelines available.

You, as a team member, must be sensitive to the client's needs, both physically and emotionally. Cultural or ethnic background must be taken into consideration and, if not accommodated, reasons given. Opportunities for discussion and explanation should be given. These guidelines apply equally to treatments and investigations.

Sometimes specific instructions are given to clients before any treatment or investigation is commenced and it is essential that the client and carers are fully conversant with all the instructions and guidance. Valuable time and resources may be wasted if instructions are not followed and unnecessary anxiety suffered.

Preparation of equipment

If you are involved in the preparation of any equipment for investigation or treatment you should be aware of how it works. Depending upon the type

Fig. 11.2 Doctor obtaining consent from a client.

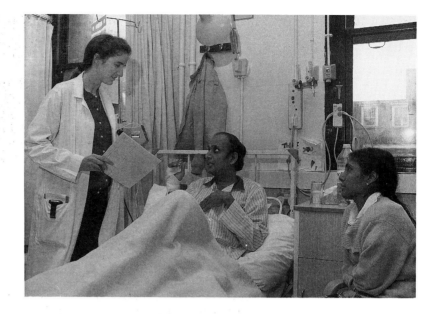

of investigation or treatment to be undertaken, the equipment will need to be clean or sterile, and certainly not damaged before use.

Activity 11.5 ■

Review all the equipment that you use. Are you aware of the recommended safe way(s) of using it and how to instruct others to prepare or use it?

■ ■

Regulations do exist to assist and protect you, your colleagues, your clients and the environment. These include the Health and Safety at Work Act 1987, the Control of Substances Hazardous to Health (1989) regulations and safety and hazard bulletins, to name a few. You also have a responsibility to ensure that any equipment that you use is safe and used for that function correctly. You must report malfunctioning equipment and your workplace should have a procedure for this.

Role of carer in investigations or treatments

During investigations or treatments your role may be to assist your client or perhaps assist your colleague(s). It is important that you understand what your role will be on each occasion. Your responsibilities will include:

■   The welfare of your client (primary responsibility).
■   Recognizing pain, distress or abnormal behaviour in your client.
■   Being aware of any *emergency procedures* that may be required.

Fig. 11.3 24-hour urine save.

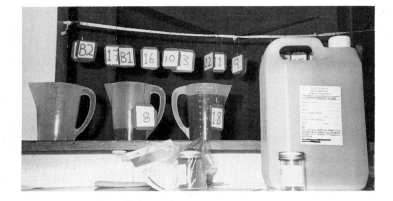

Activity 11.6   ■

Check your emergency procedures. Are you aware of where resuscitation equipment is kept and of how to use it? Where is the first aid kit? Is everything in the box that should be?

■ ■

If you are collecting specimens as part of the investigation or treatment, you must know how they are collected and in which container they should be put. Figures 11.3 and 11.4 illustrate aspects of urine collection. If in doubt ask, as incorrect preparation could lead to extra distress for the client if investigations have to be repeated. Your work area should have information on the correct procedures to be followed.

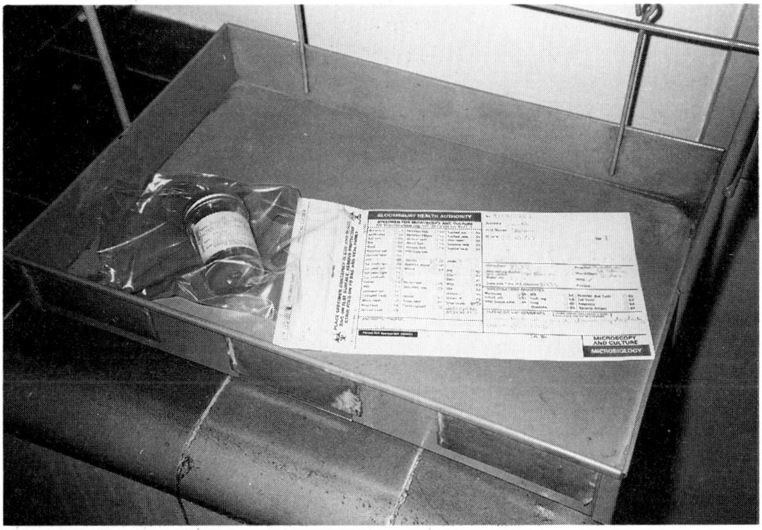

Fig. 11.4 Urine specimen in outer protective cover.

Restoration of the environment and recovery of the client

After any investigation or treatment is completed, there is the clearing up and returning of the area to normal. The client may also need observing for adverse effects of the procedure.

Restoration of the environment

It is essential to return the workplace to normal, return equipment to its storage place and dispose of items as appropriate. There may just be an emergency immediately after you finish and there is nothing worse than trying to find things when they are not in their proper place.

Storage of items must take place according to the manufacturers' and suppliers' instructions, and if there are shortages in stocks of items you should report this to the appropriate person, or take action yourself if you are the person responsible for ordering supplies.

Activity 11.7 ■

Refer back to your original list of procedures (investigations and treatments, Activity 11.2). Can you identify the observations that may need to be made on the client after those procedures; what reactions may be abnormal?

■ ■

Your list will reflect the care area in which you work. You may have to ask your colleagues to help you compile this information. Do always report items if they seem abnormal to you, it is better to be safe than sorry. The recovery of the client should be without any complications and the client should be aware of any instructions to be carried out afterwards.

Summary

For the client undergoing clinical investigations or treatments the procedure can be undertaken more smoothly if there is adequate preparation and support.

References

Boore, J.R.P. (1978) *Prescription for Recovery.* Royal College of Nursing, London.

Hayward, J. (1975) *Information – a Prescription against Pain.* Royal College of Nursing, London.

Pritchard, A.P. (1992) *The Royal Marsden Hospital Manual of Clinical Nursing Procedures*, 3rd edn. Blackwell Scientific Publications, Oxford.

Young, A.P. (1991) *Law and Professional Conduct in Nursing.* Scutari Press, London.

Further reading

Brown, J., Meikle, J. & Webb, C. (1991) Collecting midstream specimen of urine. *Nursing Times*, 27 March, **87**(13), 49–51.
Control of Substances Hazardous to Health (COSH) 1989. HMSO, London.
Health and Safety at Work Act and Amendments 1987. HMSO, London.
Jones, E. (1992) In search of a fine specimen. *Nursing Times*, 5 February, **88**(5), 62–3.

Chapter 12
Postnatal Care
Dorothy Stables

Overview

This chapter is designed to help you to care for mothers and their babies following childbirth. It includes descriptions of the changes in the mother's body and emotional state following birth. Aspects of hygiene, elimination and nutrition are covered.

The section concentrating on the baby considers the normal appearance and behaviour of the baby and how to meet the needs of the baby when the mother is unable. Psychological aspects, such as the well-being and interaction of the mother and baby, are also included along with safety, protection and security.

Key words

Puerperium, postnatal period, postnatal care of mothers, of babies, physical care, emotional care, infant feeding, artificial, breast, midwife's role, parenting.

Puerperium

Following childbirth there is a period of six weeks called the *puerperium*. Changes occur during this time in the mother's body and in the ways she feels. Ball (1989) lists these as follows:

- The reproductive organs return to their non-pregnant state.
- Other physiological changes which occurred during pregnancy are reversed.
- Lactation is established.
- The foundations of the relationship between the infant and the parents are laid.
- The mother recovers from the stresses of pregnancy and delivery and assumes responsibility for the care and nurture of her infant.

The midwife's role in the puerperium

The key professional giving care to the mother and baby during this time is the *midwife*. Two small booklets are produced by the United Kingdom

Central Council for Nursing, Midwifery and Health Visiting (UKCC) setting out the legal responsibilities and professional activities of midwives. The following brief extracts will enable you to understand the role and responsibilities of the midwife relating to the care of mothers and babies following childbirth.

Besides giving care to women during pregnancy and labour, midwives care for mothers and babies in the *postnatal period*. This is described in the UKCC (1991) handbook *Midwives' Rules* as:

> a period of not less than 10 days and not more than 28 days after the end of labour during which the continued attendance of a midwife on the mother and baby is requisite.

The midwife's activities during this time are outlined in another handbook published by the UKCC and called *A Midwife's Code of Practice* (1991). The following activities are associated with care in the postnatal period:

> to care for and monitor the progress of the mother in the postnatal period and to give all necessary advice to the mother on infant care to enable her to ensure the optimum progress of the newborn infant.

The midwife makes a full examination of all postnatal mothers in her care once or twice a day at her discretion. Your role would be to assist the midwife in the provision of quality postnatal care. You would be working under her supervision and guidance at all times but your help and assistance will be greatly appreciated. The information that follows will enable you to be competent in your practice.

Understanding the changes in the mother's body following birth

When a woman becomes pregnant most of the functions of her body alter so that her baby can grow and develop in safety. The changes in her breasts will continue during the postnatal period so that she can provide nutrition for her baby in the following months.

The uterus

During pregnancy the weight of this organ increases from around 60 grams to 1000 grams, and the length increases from around 7.5 cm to 30 cm, in order to hold the growing baby. During the six weeks following birth this organ must lose its extra tissue and revert to the size and situation it occupied before pregnancy. Most of the changes take place in the first ten days.

The obvious external sign of this change is in the vaginal loss which is heavier and lasts longer than a normal menstrual period. This loss is called *lochia* and goes through a series of colour changes as the amount of blood it contains lessens.

Did you know?

Some words in the English language look singular but are actually treated like plural words. Porridge is one such word and lochia is another. Strictly speaking we should talk about *the* lochia and *they*. The reason is similar in both examples. Porridge is short for porridge oats and lochia are made of a collection of different tissues: blood, shreds of tissue, debris from the membranes surrounding the baby and white blood cells.

As the changes in the uterus progress the lochia change colour:

- Red lochia (Lochia rubra), lasts from days 1 to 4
- Pink lochia (Lochia serosa), lasts from days 5 to 9
- White lochia (Lochia alba), lasts about another two to three weeks

Lochia have a particular odour but you should not find this offensive. As you will be involved closely with providing personal care for mothers, it is important to report to the midwife any signs of abnormal lochia either seen by you or mentioned by the mother.

Activity 12.1   ■

Make a list of some signs which may lead you to think that the lochia are abnormal.

■ ■

Your list should include the following signs, which are given with possible explanations.

- Smell offensive – may indicate an infection is present
- Heavy and red loss after the first four days – may indicate infection and be a warning of possible haemorrhage

Sanitary pads used by the mother should be saved for inspection and any blood clots passed into the toilet left for the midwife to see.

Kidneys and bladder

During pregnancy the mother increases the amount of blood circulating in her body to nourish her baby. She also accumulated more fluid in her tissues, due to the effect of hormones, and this extra fluid must now be excreted. In addition, the extra muscle tissue developed during pregnancy is now partly excreted by the kidney, by a process called autolysis. For these reasons the mother passes copious amounts of urine in the first few days after giving birth.

The mother should be encouraged to pass urine as soon as possible after the birth of the baby, preferably within the first 12 hours. Sometimes, due to the stretching of the muscles involved in giving birth and to fear of pain caused by urine passing over the graze or wound near the vaginal orifice, the mother finds it difficult to pass urine. As a further problem, she may not empty her bladder fully when she uses the toilet, passing very small amounts of urine every hour or so.

It is therefore important to observe closely both the amount of urine passed and the frequency of bedpan use or trips to the toilet. In some units mothers are encouraged to keep a chart of their fluid intake and output for the first 24 hours after normal delivery. Your role involves helping her keep her records and reporting any abnormal signs as mentioned above.

Legs

The change in the amount of fluid in the blood and tissues also increases the tendency for blood to clot. This can lead to a condition called *deep vein thrombosis* where clots form, usually in the large leg veins of the calf. The mother may complain of pain in her calves when walking. If these clots break free and travel around the body they may reach the lung and block the blood supply. She may complain of feeling faint and being unable to breathe properly. This is called a *pulmonary embolism* and the mother could die.

Reporting these signs at once to a midwife may result in a mother's life being saved. Women especially prone to this condition are those who have spent prolonged periods resting in bed and those who have had a Caesarean section to deliver their baby. Early mobilization of these mothers helps prevent the problem. Pulmonary embolism is still the most common cause of mothers dying after childbirth.

Breasts

Mothers may tell you they have painful breasts and careful questioning by you will allow sensible information to be passed on to the midwife. It is important to establish the site of the pain, whether it occurs during feeding and whether there are visible areas of redness on the skin of the breast, suggesting a possible underlying infection.

Changes in the emotional state of new mothers

Both the changes in the mother's body and her need to adapt to her new status lead many women to experience emotional ups and downs and mood swings during the first few days following birth. This is so common that it is referred to as 'fourth day blues! Green (1990) found that antenatal and labour experiences were related to postnatal mood disturbances. This was particularly so if mothers felt they had not been given sufficient information. Green also found that social and cultural aspects of mothers were not related to emotional well-being, but other studies (McIntosh,

1989) would not agree. It is probable that multiple aspects of a mother's life and health status may lead her to be unhappy following childbearing.

Support and understanding will help most women to come through their emotional turmoils. However about 10% of mothers will suffer depression serious enough to need medical referral. If a mother suffers prolonged tearful episodes or is not sleeping or eating well, is restless or seems disturbed in her relationships with baby, family or other mothers you may be the first to notice. Prompt reporting of detail to the midwife will enable adequate help to be given for this distressing state.

Postnatal care

Personal hygiene

Mothers who have had a straightforward delivery are normally fairly independent of direct care, but may need help and advice in the first few hours after the birth of their babies. Walking increases muscle tone and helps the return of blood from the legs. It also aids the passing of urine and the flow of lochia. Following normal delivery most units encourage women to walk to the bathroom and toilet within six hours. The newly delivered mother may feel a little faint the first time she walks about so it is essential that she is accompanied until she feels happy to be on her own. Remember, if the postnatal care area is away from the labour ward the mother will be unfamiliar with her surroundings and will need a guided tour and advice about the use of sitting areas and dining facilities.

It is no longer considered necessary to give each woman a form of aperient to ensure her bowels are opened. In most units the discontinuation of the routine of giving of an enema in labour has probably reduced the interference with the normal functioning of the bowel. However in the case of a mother experiencing difficulty with this function the midwife will give a mild aperient.

The mother should be advised to change her sanitary pads frequently and to keep her perineal area clean by taking a bath or shower at least once a day and, if available, sensible use of a bidet. Sometimes the midwife will carry out a procedure called vulval swabbing, especially for mothers confined to bed or those with a painful, swollen or poorly healing perineal wound.

Meeting nutritional needs

Generally most women on a postnatal unit are offered a little light refreshment such as tea and toast after the birth of their baby. They are then encouraged to rest or sleep for a while. The diet provided for new mothers should contain adequate protein to ensure tissue healing and milk production, iron and vitamins to avoid anaemia, fibre to aid bowel function and plenty of fluids.

Most hospitals provide menus for patients and most women are able to choose food that they would enjoy. Many units today cater for a multicultural population and the chef and dietitian combine their skills to provide food that is acceptable to mothers as well as containing the correct balance of nutrients.

Some mothers may not speak or read English and it may be necessary to use your ingenuity to ensure that they are provided for. It may be that a relative can help her complete the menu card during visiting, there may be a mother of the same cultural background willing to help her or the hospital may provide link workers to translate.

Activity 12.2 ■

Thinking about mothers from different cultural backgrounds, can you think of any other needs such a mother may have and other methods you could utilize to help care for her.

■ ■

Some women who have been ill during their pregnancies or who have had surgery may have special needs. These could include the provision of special diets and assistance to those unable to cut up and eat their food. The midwife looking after these mothers would advise you about any specific needs to help you provide appropriate care.

The newborn baby

Each time I see a newborn baby I feel a sense of awe at the perfection and individuality of each infant. Most babies are born after 38 to 42 weeks' gestation with no obvious abnormality and are therefore called normal. At birth they make the transition from intrauterine life to independent existence with minimal problems. This entails the following physical changes:

■ An alteration in the circulatory system to allow them to obtain oxygen by use of their lungs instead of via the placenta.
■ Inflation of the lungs to enable air to be drawn down into them and waste gases to be expelled during respiration.
■ Control of body temperature regulation.
■ Involvement of the gastrointestinal tract in the ingestion of food and excretion of wastes.
■ Activation of the immune system to combat infection.

Note that kidney function began in the uterus, where the baby passed urine into the surrounding amniotic fluid.

Recognizing the normal appearance and behaviour of the baby

The midwife has the duty to examine all babies as soon after birth as practical so that any major problems can be detected, diagnosed and treated. There are certain guidelines for deciding that a baby is normal:

- Birth weight about 3500 grams
- Length about 50 cm
- Head circumference measured at brow level will be about 35 cm
- Appearance should be rounded with a prominent abdomen
- The skin should have a pink tone, especially around the lips, whatever the ethnic background may be
- There should be good muscle tone, maintaining arms and legs in a flexed attitude in relationship to the body
- The cry should be lusty and strong, with respiratory movements continuous, if a little variable

The midwife will also examine the baby from top to toe, including the spine and genitalia, to ensure that all is well. Figure 12.1 illustrates a normal baby, born after 40 weeks gestation.

Behavioural responses to the environment around the infant and to the people caring for the infant are also important aspects of *normality*. Babies can use all their senses – hearing, sight, taste, touch and smell – and some interactions with their surroundings can be demonstrated.

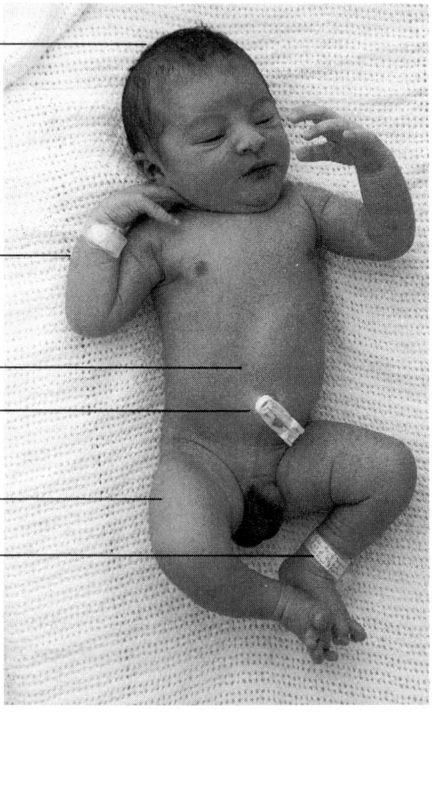

Fig. 12.1 A normal infant, born at 40 weeks.

Head large in comparison to trunk

Plump limbs with sufficient body fat

Rounded abdomen

Umbilical cord stump with clamp

Limbs flexed on trunk

Label on ankle. Note also label on right wrist

Caring for the baby in the first ten days of life when the mother is unable

Activity 12.3 ■

Take time to think about your responses to seeing and holding young babies. What is it about babies that you find appealing? You may like to consider and discuss your responses with a colleague(s).

■ ■

Your responses may include:

- The babies' facial appearances
- Their typical smell
- The feel of their bodies and their movements
- Their apparent helplessness

You might also consider these questions:

- How does the sound of their crying affect you?
- Do you enjoy looking into their eyes?
- Do you think they respond to your touch, voice or face?
- How do you feel when they hold on to your finger?

Most of us, men and women, respond with strong feelings of warmth and affection to the appearance and behaviour of new babies. This makes caring for the baby very pleasurable.

Caring for the baby's hygiene and well-being

Following the first examination of the baby after birth the midwife has a duty to examine the baby daily and to care for their safety and well-being for at least *ten days* afterwards. All mothers and babies have plans of care drawn up for them by the midwife or other appropriate professional. These plans involve mothers and yourselves as carers in all aspects of the care of the baby including bathing, feeding and interacting with the baby as a person.

One of the most important aspects of care that mothers provide for their babies is the recognition of alterations in behaviour from what they consider normal for their child. This knowledge of what is normal is acquired by the mothers in two ways. First it is the duty of the midwife and other carers to educate the mothers about infant behaviour in such a way as to create understanding and competence. Second the mothers are with their babies most of the day and soon recognize the unique responses of their own infants. No carer can afford to ignore the remarks of a mother who is anxious about her baby.

Examining the baby

If you were caring for the baby in the absence of the mother, it would be your responsibility to help detect and report deviations from the expected normal appearance and behaviour. Babies can become very ill in a short time and early detection of signs is essential.

Certain signs that may indicate illness may be seen during your care of the baby. Also a mother may tell you that she believes that there is something wrong with her baby.

The following brief *guidelines* may help you to provide valuable information for the midwife and paediatrician which could, in some circumstances, be life saving. Please note that the baby must be examined without clothing at the beginning of the cleansing and the midwife has a responsibility to carry out this examination daily. However, anyone caring for the baby may notice the following abnormalities:

- *Posture:* is the baby lying with his limbs outstretched or does he look floppy or tense?
- *Movement:* is the baby lying very still or only making feeble movements. Is he breathing normally?
- *Colour:* is the baby's skin pale, grey, blue or yellowish?
- *Blemishes:* are there any spots or pustules on the baby's skin?
- *Feeding:* is the baby taking his feeds well or refusing to feed? Is he vomiting after feeds?
- *Excretion:* have you seen evidence that the baby has passed urine and faeces in the last 24 hours?
- *Stools:* are the stools passed of normal consistency and colour for his age and feeding method?
- *Blood loss:* have you seen any signs of blood on the baby's nappy, or in his vomit or around his cord?

Bathing the baby

Each unit has procedures for the daily all over bathing of the baby and for nappy changing. You will be given practical guidance in the clinical area. There are some generalities which will enable you to adapt to new situations.

Each baby will have been identified with two labels before being removed from his mother's presence following birth. It is important that these labels remain on the baby's body whilst he remains in hospital. There have been occasional instances where mothers have taken the wrong baby home with them. If you are caring for the baby it is important that the baby's identification labels are confirmed as present, secure and correct, and if not that the appropriate professional is informed.

Another important security precaution for you to observe is never to hand the baby to anyone you do not recognize until you have positively identified them as having right of access to the baby.

Babies lose heat very quickly from their bodies and from their heads, which are large in proportion to their bodies. Also, their control of body temperature is poor in comparison with an adult and they may become chilled if they are left wet for too long. For these reasons you should ensure that the environment is warm and all equipment for bathing and changing the baby is prepared before the baby is undressed. You should also make sure your hands are washed and dried before you handle the baby.

The baby's body is washed (Fig. 12.2) and dried and, where the baby's skin is dry or sore, a topical application specified in the plan of care is used correctly. The baby is then dressed in clothes suitable for the environmental conditions.

?

Did you know?

Babies are aware of their environment and of the people caring for them. It is important that you handle the baby sensitively at all times. Also babies respond to speech and if you watch them carefully you will observe facial expressions and body movements in response to your voice. Mothers are not always aware of these facts. By your behaviour you can play an important role in helping them to relate to their babies.

Other aspects of care

Two other aspects of caring for the baby's hygiene and well-being remain. One concerns the *environment* and the other is *record keeping*. After

Fig. 12.2 Bathing a baby.

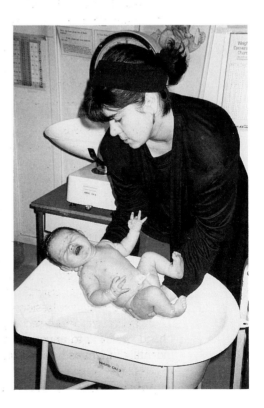

completing your care all equipment should be cleaned and stored ready for re-use and the environment should be left safe with any spillages safely cleared away. Soiled nappies, linen and other waste should be disposed of in a safe manner and place. Finally any record you are asked to make should be accurate, legible, complete and stored in the appropriate location.

Feeding and interacting with the baby

Criteria similar to those outlined for the care of the baby's hygiene and well-being apply to feeding and interacting with babies. Care given to the baby should follow the guidelines given by the midwife or other professional carer. Hands should be thoroughly washed and dried before you begin to feed or help the mother to *feed her baby*.

Artificial feeding: guidelines for care

- The correct methods of preparing and storing equipment and feed must be used (Fig. 12.3).
- The feed is made to the required quantities.
- The baby is fed in a suitable place, if possible in the mother's presence.
- The baby is fed at a pace and in a position which encourages digestion, in a manner which encourages satisfaction and at a time when she/he signals the need for food.

Fig. 12.3 Milk kitchen.

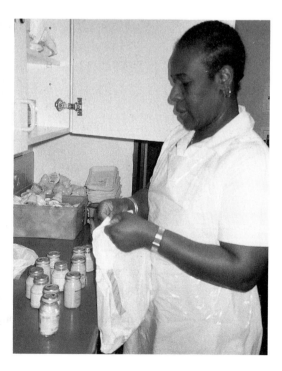

Where the baby has *problems* taking food or does not appear to be responding in the manner which is expected, *support and advice* should be sought from the midwife or other appropriate professional without delay. Where the plan of care indicates, a full accurate report of the feed and the baby's progress is made, and documents relating to the feeding process are completed. Left-over feed is disposed of in a safe manner.

Carer's role in supporting mothers in the first ten days of their babies' lives

A key role for you when working in the area of postnatal care is that of reinforcing professional advice through supporting and encouraging mothers in active parenting in the first ten days of their babies' lives. Three aspects of this will be highlighted next:

■ Assisting mothers to care for the baby's hygiene and well-being
■ Supporting mothers in feeding and interacting with their babies
■ Assisting mothers to care for babies' safety, protection and security

At all times you must be aware that the care you are giving is supervised by the midwife and any mother who is experiencing difficulty should be seen by the midwife.

Assisting mothers to care for their babies' hygiene and well-being

Most mothers, after the first postnatal day, will mainly care for their own babies. Your role will be to *assist* them in this care according to their level of skill and confidence. The above criteria of care applied to your bathing, changing and dressing the baby can be applied to the task of ensuring that the mother achieves a safe standard of care for her infant.

Supporting mothers in feeding and interacting with their babies

Whilst the guidelines on feeding babies with artificial milk will help you formulate an approach to helping the mother, many mothers choose to *breastfeed* their babies. At this point I would like to share some basic information with you to enable you to offer help to the mother with the midwife's guidance. Numerous reports and books are published about the best advice to give breastfeeding mothers. You may have read some or, indeed, have your own favourite. Those of you who have successfully breastfed a baby may have strong personal views on the best advice to give mothers.

Research into why women discontinue breastfeeding shows that one strong factor is the confusion engendered when multiple sources of advice are proffered. Even though midwives are autonomous practitioners, they follow policy guidelines of the unit so that consistent advice is given, thus helping to reduce the confusion felt by mothers. Any advice and assistance you offer should therefore be consistent with the plan developed between the midwife and the mother.

?

Did you know?

The production of breastmilk is fascinating. Here are some facts:

- Each mother manufactures the milk most suitable for her baby's age and maturity
- Breastmilk alters in its constituents as the baby grows and matures
- The quality of the milk changes as a feed progresses
- Milk is produced on a supply and demand basis – the more the baby takes, the more milk is made

Chloe Fisher (1989), a very well known expert on breastfeeding, writes:

Modern medicine entered the 'scientific' era early this century and, as a result, many practitioners came to believe that they had knowledge which would enable them to improve upon nature and they applied this belief to the management of breastfeeding.

Activity 12.4 ■

There are some well known sayings about breastfeeding with which you may be familiar. Make a list of any you know.

■ ■

Your list may include:

(1) Babies should be put to the breast every four hours.
(2) Feeds should last for three minutes a side on the first day and then be increased until ten minutes a side are given.
(3) Babies who appear dissatisfied after a feed should be given a top-up feed of modified cows' milk.
(4) Both breasts should be offered at each feed.
(5) Breastmilk may be too watery for the baby so top-up feeds may be necessary.
(6) Women with small breasts cannot make sufficient milk.
(7) Women with flat nipples cannot breastfeed.

You may well be able to add to this list from your personal knowledge and experience. *None of the above tenets is now held by experienced carers.*
For you to help mothers to breastfeed their babies, good technique

cannot be taught in a text book. It is best acquired by observation and experience. There is a very good booklet, *Successful Breastfeeding*, by the Royal College of Midwives (1988), which will help you to understand the advice given to mothers by midwives.

Modern practice is underpinned by the following:

- The baby is put to the breast as often as he wants for as long as he wants.
- Top-up feeds are not generally given as the decrease in suckling brought about by excess milk will only result in a fall in milk production, creating a vicious circle of artificial feeding and reduced production of breastmilk and the end result is usually discontinuation of breastfeeding and a mother who may feel a failure.

Practical help for the mother

If you are assisting to prepare for breastfeeding the following tips are helpful:

Hygiene

The midwife will advise the mother to wash her breasts daily. It is not thought necessary to undergo elaborate bathing and breast preparation before each feed. Mothers are encouraged to wear a supporting brassiere and to use pads inside the cups if their breasts leak between feeds.

Positioning of the mother

Mothers may breastfeed their babies lying down or sitting up. In both positions the mother should feel physically comfortable so that she can concentrate on feeding the baby.

Positioning the baby

The baby needs to be supported with his body turned towards the mother's breast and his mouth opposite the mother's nipples (Fig. 12.4). His neck should be slightly extended. Usually the midwife will want to supervise any mother who is having difficulty breastfeeding and she will appreciate any information about such mothers that you become aware of during your care.

Parent and baby interaction

Many young mothers in Britain, especially those of the indigenous population, have little or no contact with small babies before the birth of their own child. Families are now smaller and brothers and sisters may not live close by. An important role for those providing care in the early days is to help mothers *relate* to their babies. In fact, midwives now emphasize the

Fig. 12.4 Breastfeeding.

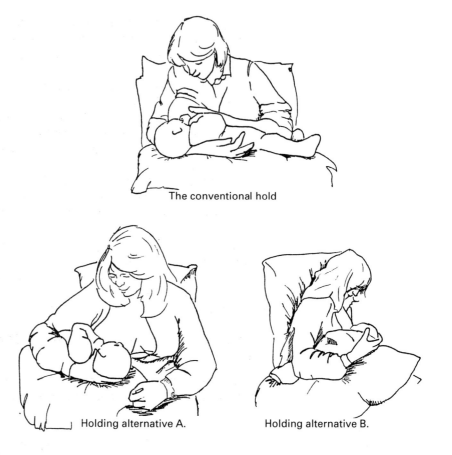

The conventional hold

Holding alternative A.   Holding alternative B.

importance of the role of the father and consider themselves to be family-centred professionals.

As already indicated, babies respond to their *environment* and to the people around them. But young parents may not realize this. Indeed, mothers may be so anxious about the physical care and feeding of their babies that relationships take second place.

Babies are born with their *senses* quite well developed. They can see quite well and their best focus is about 9 inches (23 cm), which allows them to see their mother's face clearly when held in the usual breastfeeding position. They can hear clearly and respond by moving their heads in the direction of the noise, especially speech. They synchronize their body movements with speech.

They can soon discriminate their mother's breastmilk smell from the milk of other women and will turn towards that smell and try to suckle from the source. They can also distinguish taste and pull disgusted faces if bitter tastes, such as some medicines, are given to them.

Babies can feel cold and pain and should be handled carefully. Indeed, they respond to physical discomfort with vigorous crying.

Many parents have no knowledge of their infant's wide range of behaviour. Research has shown that parenting skills are improved when the following facts are made available to them:

■ Touch and eye contact are very important points in any relationship and it is best if, following delivery, parents are given time to be alone together with their baby. The midwife will encourage the mother to feed her baby. Close physical and eye contact should be encouraged.
■ Parents should smile at and talk to the baby when he is awake and alert (Fig. 12.5).
■ Some mothers take longer than others to relate to their babies and it's important that those in whom strong feelings of affection take a while to blossom should be reassured that they are not abnormal.

However, if you notice any mother or father treating their baby roughly or speaking about their baby in a negative way you should immediately notify the midwife. The mother may be disturbed emotionally or the child might be at risk of abuse and your prompt action may help the family to receive the necessary help for them to adjust to their baby.

Assisting mothers to care for babies' safety, protection and security

All the above information, when put together, can help the mother develop sensible and safe approaches to the care of her baby. The advice to carers

Fig. 12.5 Mother and baby interaction.

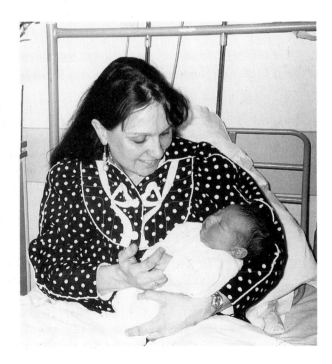

about babies' labels, not handing the baby to unidentified people, caring for the environment, and the hygiene and safe handling of the baby can be reinforced by you so that the chances of danger to the baby are kept to a minimum.

Summary

Following childbirth there is a period of *six weeks* called the *puerperium*. Physical and psychological changes occur during this time. The key professional giving care to the mother and baby during this time is the *midwife*. Her duties include caring for and monitoring the progress of the mother in the postnatal period and giving all necessary advice to the mother on infant care to enable optimum progress of the newborn infant. The midwife makes a full examination of all postnatal mothers and their babies once or twice daily for the first *ten days* after birth at her discretion.

Mothers who have had a straightforward delivery are normally fairly independent of direct care, but may need help and advice in the first few hours after the birth of their babies.

All mothers and babies have *plans of care* drawn up for them by the midwife or other appropriate professional. These plans involve mothers and yourselves as *carers* in all aspects of care of the baby including bathing, feeding and interacting with the baby as a person.

Women who have been ill during their pregnancies or who have had surgery may have *special needs*, for example the provision of special diets and temporary assistance in cutting up and eating their food. The midwife looking after these mothers would advise you about any specific needs to enable you to help provide care.

Your role in caring for mothers and their babies in the postnatal period would be to *assist the midwife*. You would be working under her supervision and guidance at all times but your help and assistance will be greatly appreciated. Care will include:

- Enabling mothers to maintain their personal hygiene and assisting mothers to access and use toilet facilities.
- Enabling mothers to choose appropriate food and drink and assisting mothers with eating and drinking when necessary.
- Supporting mothers in feeding and interacting with their babies.
- Caring for the baby in the first ten days of life when the mother is unable.
- Assisting mothers to care for their babies' hygiene and well-being.
- Assisting mothers to care for babies' safety, protection and security.

References

Ball, J.A. (1989) Physiology, psychology and management of the puerperium. In *Myles Textbook for Midwives* 11th edn (Ed. by V.R. Bennett & L.L. Brown) Churchill Livingstone, Edinburgh.

Fisher, C. (1989) Feeding. In *Myles Textbook for Midwives*, 11th edn (Ed. by V.R. Bennett & L.K. Brown). Churchill Livingstone, Edinburgh.

Green, J.M. (1990) Who is unhappy after childbirth? Antenatal and intrapartum correlates from a prospective society. *Journal of Reproductive and Infant Psychology*, **8**(3), 175–84.

McIntosh, J. (1989) Models of childbirth and social class: a study of 80 working class primigravidae. In *Midwives, Research and Childbirth*, Vol. 1 (Ed. by S. Robinson and A. Thomson). Chapman and Hall, London.

Royal College of Midwives (1991) *Successful Breastfeeding*, 2nd edn. Churchill Livingstone, Edinburgh.

UKCC (1991) *A Midwife's Code of Practice*. United Kingdom Central Council for Nursing, Midwifery and Health Visiting, London.

UKCC (1991), *Midwives' rules*. United Kingdom Central Council for Nursing, Midwifery and Health Visiting, London.

Further reading

Trevellyan, J. & Fardell, J. (1992) Care of the Mother and Newborn. Macmillan, London.

Laryea, M. (1984) *Postnatal Care: The Midwife's Role*. Churchill Livingstone, Edinburgh.

Ball, J.A. (1986) *Reactions to Motherhood: The Role of Postnatal Care*. Cambridge University Press, Cambridge.

Prince, J. & Adam, M.E. (1987) *The Psychology of Childbirth*. Churchill Livingstone, Edinburgh.

Klaus, M.H. & Kennel, J.H. (1982) *Parent–Infant Bonding*. Mosby, St Louis.

Minchin, M. (1989) *Breast Feeding Matters*. Allen and Unwin, Australia.

Renfrew, M., Fisher, C. & Arms, S. (1990) *Best Feeding: Getting Breast Feeding Right for You*. Celestial Arts, Berkeley, USA.

Chapter 13
Care of the Young Child
Lisa S. Whiting

Overview

In this chapter we will consider the principles of care of the child in hospital. Attention will be paid to the effects of hospitalization, the role of the family, the importance of play and the maintenance of a safe environment. Psychological care will be considered throughout, but specific physical care will not be included since it is beyond the scope of this chapter.

Key words

Child, family, separation, partnership, play, communication, safety, child abuse.

Helping child and family to adapt to hospitalization

Effects of separation

As a *child* you may have been in hospital and have memories of how it felt to be *separated* from *family*, friends, home and toys. As carers our prime concern with children is to understand the effects of separation and how these may be minimized. John Bowlby (1951), an eminent psychiatrist, who specialized in child psychology, believed that

> the infant and young child should experience a warm, intimate, and continuous relationship with his mother (or permanent mother-substitute) in which both find satisfaction and enjoyment.

When Bowlby was conducting his work, it was common practice for children in hospital to be separated from their families and for visiting to be very restricted, for example once a week, and parents only. This was thought to be advantageous as the children frequently became distressed when their parents left. Today, families are encouraged to spend as much time together with their child as possible (Fig. 13.1). Nevertheless parental separation does still occur and its effect on the child should be understood.

Research by James Robertson (1958), a social worker, identified stages

Fig. 13.1 Mother and son awaiting tests in hospital.

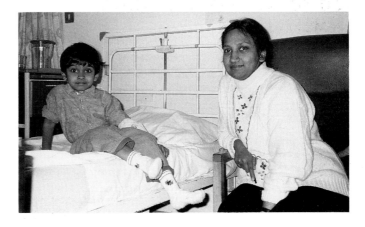

of adjustment that young children exhibit when separated from their families. He suggested that the child between six months and four years of age is particularly vulnerable to the effects of separation and hospitalization:

> If at this crucial stage in his development, when he has such a possessive and passionate need for his mother, and he is blindly trustful of his parents, he is admitted alone to hospital, he experiences a serious failure of that environment of love and security hitherto provided by his family and which we know to be a necessary experience if he is to be a loving, secure and trustful person in later life.

The effects of separation, as identified by Robertson, are given below. Such reactions may be seen even when the period of separation is brief.

Protest

■ The child is grief-stricken, calling constantly for the parent(s). As the young child lives in the present he may feel deserted by parents.
■ The child is likely to reject the hospital carer and may become openly hostile.

Despair

■ The child sinks into apparent depression, becoming quiet, apathetic and withdrawn, mourning for the lost parent(s).
■ The child may adopt self-comforting behaviours, such as thumb-sucking, and may regress developmentally, for example in potty training, play activities or language.
■ The child may exhibit behavioural difficulties and sleep problems.
■ When parents visit, the child may become upset.

Denial

- The child no longer appears depressed and shows interest in the immediate surroundings. The child may now repress all feelings for the parent(s).
- If the child has a prolonged hospital stay, he may settle into the routine and way of life. This may lead to long-term emotional disturbances.
- The child might also become the 'pet' of carers, receiving 'special' attention and care.

Although it is generally agreed that young children are most susceptible to the effects of separation and hospitalization, children of any age who require repeated admissions, or whose condition necessitates a single protracted period in hospital, are also at risk (Bowlby, 1969; Shannon *et al.*, 1984).

Take some time to observe children in your work area. Do any of them exhibit any signs of the behaviours identified above?

Activity 13.1 ■■■■■■■■■■■■■■■■■■■■■■■■

 Many other problems are associated with hospitalization of children. Take time to consider other effects on the child, the parents, brothers and/or sisters (siblings) and make a list of points.

■■■■■■■■■■■■■■■■■■■■■■■■■■■■■■

Your list may include all or some of the following:

Effects on the child

- Disruption of home routine, particularly important for the very young child.
- The child may become very confused, fearful of being hurt, and may then revert to baby-like behaviour which is known as regression.
- Schoolwork may be neglected.
- The child may not sleep properly.

Effects on the parents

- They may feel the need to be in two places at once, i.e. with their child and at home with the rest of the family.
- Financial problems may arise, e.g. loss of earnings or extra expenses incurred for travelling.
- Parents may become physically and emotionally exhausted.

■ *Bonding* between baby and parents may be reduced.
■ The whole family may be thrown into 'crisis'.

Effects on the siblings

■ Siblings may express a number of feelings:
   Guilt that they may somehow have caused the child's illness;
   Resentment and jealousy that they are receiving less attention than the sick child;
   Anger that they are not kept informed of the child's illness or invited to participate in the events of care.

In recognition of these potentially damaging effects upon the child and family, the Ministry of Health report, as long ago as 1959, recommended that

the child should not be admitted to hospital if it can possibly be avoided.

The degree to which a young child becomes disturbed due to separation depends on a number of factors now identified:

■ The child's age and stage of development.
■ The nature of the child/parent relationship.
■ The frequency of previous separations. The child who has been in hospital on a number of previous occasions may appear to adapt to the next admission more easily than the child who has never been away from parents or stayed away from home overnight. It is important to remember, however, that appearances may be deceptive. The quiet, composed child may be experiencing inner turmoil.
■ The preparation that the child received prior to admission. It may be well-nigh impossible to prepare the child admitted as a result of sudden illness or accident. However, for the child whose admission is planned, both physical and psychological preparation can be made. This preparation will be discussed later.
■ The role of parents while the child is in hospital. Continuous contact with parents during the child's stay is vital. If one parent can be resident, this will help to maintain security and stability for the child.
■ The amount of sensory stimulation that the child receives. The provision of appropriate play materials, suitable for the child's developmental age, is essential.
■ The parents' response to changed events and routine. Children are particularly receptive to the way their parents react, and this can have an important influence on the experience of being in hospital.

These factors affect the child while in hospital, but it is equally important to remember that they will also affect the child's behaviour after they return home.

Easing the effects of separation

Activity 13.2 ■

 We have identified the effects of hospitalization on both the child and family. It is becoming clear that some of these effects need to be minimized as far as possible. Either by yourself or with a group of colleagues, make a list of some actions that could be taken to reduce some of these problems.

■ ■

Some of your solutions may include the following:

- Encourage parent(s) to spend as much time as possible with their child. There can be no doubt that illness makes the child more dependent and increases the need for close contact with the family, in particular with the mother. Where possible the parent(s) should be offered the opportunity to be resident with their child, but pressure should not be applied.
- Encourage the whole family to participate in the child's care, provided they are willing and happy to do so and have received any necessary instruction.
- As carers we can help by staying with the child when the parent(s) are not visiting. The use of diversional play can be very valuable, as can cuddling and comforting the child.
- Preserve, as far as possible, the child's home routine, such as bedtime, bath time, story time.
- Ask parents to bring the child's usual and favourite toys/comforters. Parents may feel embarrassed that their four- or five-year-old still has a dummy; reassurance needs to be given that this is not the time to remove the comforter; in fact it may be of more help than usual.
- Encourage siblings to visit and be involved in care. Adolescents may particularly value seeing their friends and peers.
- Share information with the whole family about the child's care and management on a regular basis. Questions should be answered and information expressed in understandable terms. Strategies employed to reduce parental anxiety can be expected to have both direct and indirect benefits for the child.
- Psychological preparation of the child for procedures, for example the taking of blood, administration of drugs or an operation, should be carried out in a similar manner to that previously discussed in connection with adult clients in Chapter 11.
- Keep the number of carers involved in the child's care to a minimum to avoid the confusion created by too many strangers and, more important, to give the family ample opportunity to build and preserve relationships.
- Take time to listen and talk with the family.

It is clear that a period in hospital can have a profound effect upon the psychological welfare of the child. It is therefore our responsibility to attempt to minimize problems and to work towards returning the child to their home environment and family as soon as possible. It may then be that the whole experience will be one of positive learning for both child and family.

Care in partnership with the family

The involvement of the family in care of the child in hospital has already been mentioned. As this is such an important feature of care we will now explore it in more detail.

The *Concise Oxford Dictionary* describes the family as a

Set of parents and children, or of relations, living together or not.

Sociologists have attempted to define the term family, but definitions tend to vary tremendously. However, the inclusion of children appears a common thread. Murdock (1965) describes the family as being a social group who live together. The group includes male and female adults, two of whom maintain a socially approved sexual relationship and have one or more children. Bond & Bond (1986) offer the view that the family is a universal institution taking many forms within one culture and between different cultures.

Almost all of us have an in-depth knowledge and closeness with at least one family, and this may influence our personal opinions of what constitutes a family. You may have noticed how your own particular family differs in its organizational structure from those of your friends. In some families the mother is the central figure – sociologists call this the *matriarchal family* – while other families are father-centred and this is the *patriarchal family*. Some families are neither mother nor father centred and some are single parent families.

Activity 13.3   ■

Consider families which you know and try to identify the description given above which best fits them.

■ ■

The family has become idealized within British culture, being seen as valuable, good and worthwhile. Politicians have extolled the virtues of the family. Others, such as Barrett & McIntosh (1982), have echoed this view saying that the family is the most appropriate institution in which to rear children and help them to become 'competent and secure, stable and self-sufficient'.

It is, therefore, no surprise that the concept of the British family is one of *happiness* revolving round the image of two married parents who share a family home with their children. Today, however, this is not always the case. Although the family may be the source of happy and positive experiences, it can also be the cause of negative experiences. All families at some time will face problems and go through phases of crisis and turmoil.

Changes in society influence family life and values and the changes today are many, rapid, varied and far-reaching. Demographic trends indicate that people tend to have fewer children than they did 50 years ago. Contraception is widely available and practised and termination of pregnancy is legal. Families are subjected to a number of social pressures, such as maintaining a high standard of living. As a result many women return to work after the birth of their children in order to contribute to family finances.

Alterations in lifestyle also include rising unemployment; more adults choose to cohabit rather than marry; increasing divorce rates and re-marriages lead to mixings of partners and their children. Finally, growing numbers of different ethnic groups are represented in our society, all of whom have differing values and cultures.

A fair conclusion would be that the classic image of Mr and Mrs Average with their two children – the family – may be difficult to find! The acceptance and reasonable understanding of different family structures and cultures is vital if we, as carers, are to work in partnership with *the whole family*.

Activity 13.4 ■

From your experience, make a list of the different family structures that you have encountered as part of your work.

■ ■

Your list may be very extensive. Here are some possibilities:

- Two parents and their children, all from the same cultural background
- Two parents and their children, parents from different cultural backgrounds
- A one-parent family, as a result of:
    divorce/separation
    death of one partner
    single, relationship with partner never fully established
- Parents who have adopted children from the same or a different cultural background
- Families with their own children and others who are fostered
- Two lesbians or homosexuals who may have children from previous marriages

For many people in our society, the immediate nuclear family is

Fig. 13.2 Mother and daughter in hospital.

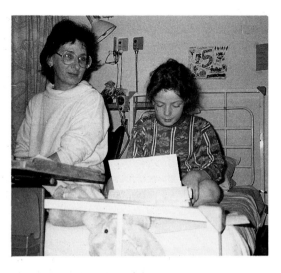

primarily responsible for the child's upbringing. This may be because people are mobile and tend to move to different geographical locations in seeking/changing employment, and relatives are no longer close at hand. Conversely, for others, particularly ethnic minority groups, the extended family (grandparents, aunts, uncles, cousins) often plays an important role in the early development and care of the child (Fig. 13.2).

Family reactions to the hospitalization of their child

Approximately one million children are admitted to hospital in England each year (Caring for Children in the Health Services, 1987). To many families this event is the cause of great stress. For us, the carers, it is sometimes difficult to appreciate the anxiety parents experience. This may be particularly so if the child has been admitted for what seems to be a relatively *minor* treatment. However, it seems that parents' reactions and the degree of stress experienced vary little regardless of the child's diagnosis or the severity of the illness. The child is precious beyond measure to parents and no illness or treatment is small or unimportant. If the child is very sick the parents' reactions become more intense and persistent.

Activity 13.5 ■

Make a note of how you think parents may react to their child's hospitalization.

■ ■

You may have identified some of the following emotions:

- *Disbelief*, especially if the illness is sudden.
- *Guilt:* the parent(s) may search for self-blame. They may ask 'Why is our child ill? Was it something we did?'
- *Anger:* parents may vent angry feelings towards those caring for their child.
- *Fear/anxiety* may be directly related to the child's illness, or to the investigations/treatment to be carried out.
- *Frustration* can arise because the parent is given insufficient information about the child's illness and they may not understand what they are expected to do while their child is in hospital.
- *Depression* sometimes occurs while the child is in hospital, but can also cause problems following discharge. Parents may comment that they feel mentally and physically exhausted once the child is home. Their feelings may also be due to the child's long-term prognosis, any negative effects induced by the hospital stay and financial problems that may have arisen as a result.

Encouraging the family to become involved in the child's care

The family, and in particular the parents, may see the child's hospital stay as a very traumatic experience. Some of these feelings can be alleviated by encouraging them to be involved in the child's care.

When referring to family participation we think primarily of *parents*, but any member who plays a significant role in the child's upbringing may be involved. Encouraging siblings to participate helps to deal with some of the negative reactions which we described earlier, and also helps to maintain the family unit. *Partnership with the family* should be the focus of all the care given to the child in hospital.

Activity 13.6 ■

Make some notes about how you think you could encourage the family to participate in their child's care.

■ ■

Your notes may include some of the following points:

Encouragement

A parent may become extremely distressed when someone else is caring for their child. Encouraging one or more family members to spend as much time as possible with the child provides opportunity for them to be involved in planning and giving care and possibly hastens the child's recovery.

Families may carry out the child's washing and feeding or wish to be involved in areas of care new to them. There is no reason why the family should not take over responsibility for any aspect of their child's care provided they are happy to do so and they receive appropriate preparation and support. However, not all families feel comfortable taking this kind of responsibility so it is important not to pressurize them.

Recognizing parents as experts

Some families will be highly skilled in caring for their child, particularly if the child has a chronic disease. All parents are able to offer valuable advice and information about their child's normal home routine and lifestyle.

Providing support

This involves willingness to listen and respond to the family's concerns and anxieties. This may help parents to accept their own feelings towards their sick child. Support could also be more practical help, such as offering to sit and cuddle the child while the parent goes for a cup of tea.

Offering advice

This may be advice about how to carry out any aspect of the child's care. Alternatively, it may be suggesting to other relatives how they might help, for example caring for other children at home or doing household chores, so that parents are relieved of some of these burdens.

Accepting family cultural, socio-economic and ethnic values

The parents may wish to introduce others they regard as important to their child's care, for example a representative of their religious faith or a practitioner of a complementary therapy such as massage. Medical advice may need to be sought for the latter.

Providing advice and information

If the parents are fully aware of the child's illness and the planned management, so much anxiety is relieved. The sick child, if old enough, and other family members may need to be involved in these discussions. Explanations of how siblings may react to the child's hospitalization will help parents to appreciate the need to involve them in the care.

Caring team

The child should be cared for by as few people as possible to give continuity of care and to give the parents the opportunity to build relationships, confidence and a sense of control, making them feel part of the team.

The multidisciplinary team

Other personnel may be involved in the child's care, such as doctors, social workers, speech therapists, physiotherapists, and it is important that a team approach is employed and that individuals do not operate in isolation.

To summarize, the following three points encapsulate the discussion:

■ Ask the family for which aspects of care they would like to take responsibility
■ Build the family's confidence by giving reassurance and information
■ Give the family support and encouragement when they are giving care

Role of the carer

Now a word about carers. Although when caring for children the client/carer relationship is extended due to the presence of the family, the responsibility for care still lies with the registered practitioner whom you are assisting. Initially you may find it stressful working closely with the family, and may even feel that you are under their scrutiny – indeed those of you who are parents may easily appreciate the family's viewpoint in this matter. However, this is something that you will become used to in time – remember caring for the child in partnership with the family can greatly enhance the child's recovery.

The child and play

'Play is an essential part of *every* child's life and vital to the process of human development' (National Voluntary Council for Children's Play, 1992). As the child's life needs to progress as normally as possible, we will examine the stages and types of play, the provision of play for the child in hospital and how play can be used as a part of care.

Stages of play

Play has many functions and purposes. Individual children play in different ways – some quietly, others noisily and actively. Despite these apparent differences, children generally adopt styles of play according to their age.

■ *Solitary play* is adopted by young children up to approximately two years of age (Fig. 13.3). They prefer to play alone, although like to have a parent nearby. At this stage repetition is important – you may have seen a young child deriving great amusement from repeatedly throwing a toy or teddy out of the cot.
■ *Parallel play:* children between three and four years of age enjoy playing alongside each other. They may briefly interact, perhaps to show one another an interesting object, but each child continues to play independently for most of the time.
■ *Social play:* at approximately four years of age the child has usually begun to play with others in small groups of perhaps two, three or

Fig. 13.3 Toddler at play.

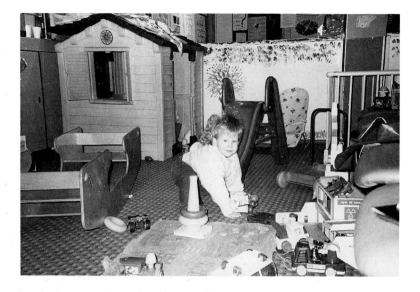

four. At this stage children are learning to share and interact with others but they will still use solitary and parallel play.

Types of play

There are many types of play, all of which develop particular skills in the child. Ideally, the child should have the opportunity to participate in the different types throughout childhood. Examples include:

- Active play
- Constructive play
- Social play
- Games with rules

- Exploratory play
- Make-believe play
- Problem-solving play
- Hobbies

Role of the carer

Children need adults to help them to play and to provide them with suitable play materials. However, it is important not to be too directive, and to allow the child to use their imagination. Sometimes one can feel lost and not know *how to play* with children. The following suggestions may help:

- Make yourself comfortable and sit at the child's level.
- Introduce the child to others so that they have the opportunity to play together. This is particularly important for those who are four years of age and over.
- Give praise and encouragement to the child if they accomplish something well, for example a two-year-old completing a simple jig-saw puzzle. At the same time, try not to reinforce negative behaviour

such as a child hitting another with a toy hammer! The most suitable action is to tell the child kindly but firmly that this is wrong. It may be necessary to physically separate the children and divert their attentions with other games.

■ Join in with the child's play, for example board games, role play, *hospital play*.

■ Ensure that all children in your care have equal opportunities to participate in play, irrespective of age, culture or disability.

■ At all times consider the safety of children whilst they are at play. This includes factors such as adequate supervision and the provision of toys that conform to British and European standards.

■ Respect the family's cultural, religious and social beliefs in the course of play.

Activity 13.7   ■

What play facilities/materials would you suggest as appropriate for children of the following ages? Give two examples for each age group.

Birth–6 months	3–5 years
6 months–1 year	5–7 years
1–2 years	8–12 years
2–3 years	12 years onwards

■ ■

Here are a few suggestions:

Birth to six months

Babies of this age like colourful objects they can watch and listen to such as mobiles, rattles, mirrors and soft cuddly toys. They also enjoy activities such as *finger play*.

Six months to one year of age

These babies will be becoming more inquisitive and will need toys that give them the opportunity to develop skills. Examples include activity centres and mats, building bricks, toy telephone, and they usually love playing in the bath with buckets or squeezy toys.

One to two years of age

The child at this age has begun to explore – many are very mobile. Suitable play materials include push-along toys, posting boxes, toys that they sit and ride on, simple jig-saws and stacking toys.

Two to three years of age

Children of this age particularly enjoy make-believe play and dressing-up. Appropriate play materials would include old clothes, dolls, domestic equipment like saucepans, tea sets, large nuts and bolts, sandpit with bucket and spade. At the same time the child has developed more advanced motor movement, so objects like large beads to make a necklace, paints and brushes, climbing frames and swings will also be popular.

Three to five years of age

This group is acquiring new skills very rapidly. They enjoy construction toys, larger jig-saws, cutting-out (with blunt scissors), making collages, playing doctors and nurses, play-dough, finger-painting, wendy houses.

Five to seven years of age

Children of this age like to make things, so simple embroidery, cookery, basic woodwork, for example, may be suitable. They also enjoy more active games like football and skipping.

Eight to twelve years of age

More complex toys that require a certain amount of skill can now be introduced, such as computer and board games. They may also, by now, have a number of hobbies: cooking, swimming, horse riding, to name a few.

Twelve years onwards

This age group is more interested in pursuing individual interests and hobbies, so it is important to identify what these are. Most common examples include listening to music, talking with friends, sport activities and computer games.

The above are just a few ideas that you may find helpful in your work. Most importantly, it is essential to identify the child's individual interests and seek to accommodate these.

Play for the child in hospital

Play for the child in hospital 'is one of the few elements of normal life in an abnormal situation' (Play in Hospital Liaison Committee, 1990). It should be available to all children, in whichever department they are being cared for including casualty and out-patient departments, because it fulfils so many vital functions.

Play promotes continuation of growth and development and helps to minimize regression. It can help the child to deal with the stress of the situation and gives the child opportunity to express feelings and emotions. By reducing anxiety it can speed recovery and therefore shorten the hospital stay.

It can form excellent diversional therapy, occupy the child and prevent or relieve boredom. Play can enable children to relate to staff, and prepare children both for admission and for medical procedures, such as blood tests, removal of a plaster of Paris cast and surgery. It may also reduce parental anxiety as it allows the family to participate in some of the child's normal activities.

We have already identified that when children are ill and in hospital some aspects of their development may regress. For this same reason, children may choose to play with toys which make them feel comfortable and secure, but are more suited to a younger age group. In the circumstances concentration span may be limited and interest in a particular toy also, so a variety of play materials should be available. Observation of the child at play is important and may give the first indication of emotional upset or regression. As carers we may be the first to notice these changes.

All children in hospital should be encouraged to play in some form, however sick or disabled they may be. However, it is important to recognize that the illness or necessary treatment may limit both the child's capacity for and interest in play.

Using play to prepare a child for medical procedures

Play can also be used to help prepare children for medical procedures such as an operation. Your work area may have a *hospital corner* which has a stock of uniforms, bandages, stethoscopes and books. Children may ask you to participate in their hospital play, for example to be a patient or to help bandage teddy's arm.

Let us consider an example of using play towards a child's treatment.

Activity 13.8 ■

Leroy is five years old and has been admitted to hospital for removal of his adenoids and tonsils. Make some notes to cover how you think play therapy could be used to help prepare him for his operation

■ ■

Your notes may include some of the following points:

■ Identify Leroy's present level of knowledge. What does he know about his forthcoming operation? Has he been in hospital before? What have his parents told him and what toys or books have they used to help prepare him for the admission and the surgery.
■ Establish how Leroy feels about his operation. Is he frightened, or is he calm and relaxed? This will influence the amount and intensity of preparation required.

When these questions have been answered, Leroy's knowledge can be built upon during the pre-operative period. A number of methods can be used to help prepare Leroy for this operation:

■ Books telling stories about children coming into hospital can be read to him and he may enjoy looking at the pictures. (Suitable books are listed in the Further reading section at the end of this chapter.) Booklets and photograph albums may be available to explain procedures and care for children in your specific area.

■ Some clinical areas have videos depicting children going to theatre for particular operations. If available, these may prove very useful, along with someone available to answer Leroy's and his parents' questions.

■ Leroy's favourite toys may be included in the preparation, particularly if they are going to accompany him to theatre. Leroy may like teddy to be a patient too and so the opportunity exists for Leroy to see and hear what will happen when he is prepared for operation by demonstrating and explaining using teddy. Then when Leroy goes for his operation teddy can go too.

Clear, truthful explanations appropriate to Leroy's level of understanding are essential. It is particularly important to explain to Leroy when he will go home and to discuss any unpleasant side effects that he may experience afterwards, such as a sore throat. To be truthful is to preserve the child's trust. You may find that both child and parent(s) need the information repeated a number of times to give them a chance to absorb what is being said.

Family members should be involved in all aspects of the child's preparation. You may find that little preparation is required for some children going to theatre, for others more time and a combination of techniques may be appropriate.

Clearly these points could easily be adapted to help prepare children who are to undergo other medical procedures and treatments, such as insertion of infusions, physiotherapy, application of plaster splints, speech therapy. The planned psychological preparation of a child is not always successful, but it does help allay the anxiety in many children and their parents.

Other functions of play

Play has a number of other functions, for example children may use it to express their emotions. A child who has suffered abuse may use a doll or teddy to role play experiences; a teenager who is going through an emotional crisis may express feelings in drawings or poetry. For this reason, it is vital that we observe and listen to children at play and take their views and actions seriously. If you are concerned or worried about the significance of a child's play, do not hesitate to convey this to a senior member of staff.

Using play to aid a child's care and management

Finally we can also incorporate play into a child's care and management. For example, Emma is five years of age and has cystic fibrosis and needs to practise deep breathing exercises to help improve her lung function. This could be made more fun by encouraging her to blow bubbles. Likewise, James has cerebral palsy and the fine movement and coordination of his fingers are poor, so the use of jigsaw puzzles may prove beneficial. Or, Gemma, one year old, requires physiotherapy for her legs; toys may divert her attention whilst she is undergoing her exercises.

We see that play is vital to the growth and development of the child, and that it has a particularly significant role for those in hospital. It is our responsibility to ensure that all children in our care have the opportunity to experience a variety of play activities appropriate to their individual needs.

Maintaining a safe environment for the child in hospital

The last part of this chapter is devoted to issues concerned with child safety. Sadly accidents create the need for a considerable number of child admissions to hospital and, more sadly, accidents do happen in hospital. Although all references to safety throughout this book apply equally to the care of children, as a conclusion we will explore important *safety* aspects specific to children.

Accidents

Over the last 20 years, accidents have emerged as *the* major health problem for children aged between one and 14 years. 'Children's accidents result in 700 deaths, 120 000 hospital admissions and about 2 million casualty department attendances in England and Wales *every year*' (Child Accident Prevention Trust, 1989). Thus, accidents are clearly a significant cause of distress for both the child and family. You will probably be involved in the care of children who have been admitted to hospital as a result of an accident – perhaps due to a fall, the inhalation or swallowing of a foreign body or a scald.

A significant number of accidents (three-quarters of a million each year) occur in the home environment (Child Accident Prevention Trust, 1989). However, it could be argued that there are far more hazards in hospital than in the child's home, so extra precautions need to be taken to ensure that the environment is as safe as possible. Until recently, the problem of accidents to children in hospital has received little attention, but Levene & Bonfield (1991) found in their research that 781 accidents occurred in the eight hospitals studied over an 18-month period. Most of these involved boys, aged three to five years, the most common incidents being falls from a height, slipping and striking accidents.

Environmental hazards in hospital

We will now consider some of the environmental hazards. It is important to remember that hospital is a strange environment for the child and family, so this alone may increase the risk of accidents.

Activity 13.9 ■

 Look around your clinical area and make a list of the environmental hazards that could cause accidental injury to a child.

■ ■

No doubt you will have many ideas; here are a few suggestions:

- Hot drinks left on bedside lockers
- Toys: a toddler or child may inhale or swallow small parts of toys and children may trip over toys
- Equipment such as intravenous infusion pumps: a young child may walk into the pump and its stand; a child may play with the plug/plug socket/buttons of the infusion pump
- Sharp objects not correctly disposed of
- Unattended drug trolley
- Ward door left open: all clinical areas should have child safety gates/ doors
- Spillages on floors causing a parent or child to slip
- Uniform accessories of carers, such as badges with sharp edges (these may be harmful when cuddling a child), or scissors that can easily be pulled from your pocket
- Radiators could be a potential cause of burns; all should have radiator guards
- Windows are particularly hazardous if your clinical area is not on the ground floor; window guards and child safety locks are essential

Safety precautions in hospital

Apart from environmental factors, accidents can occur if hospital procedures or protocol are not strictly adhered to. No doubt we have all read newspaper articles about patients who have had the wrong surgery or drugs. Young children are perhaps even more at risk, since their verbal communication skills are limited. The following are examples of how we can all work towards ensuring that the child's planned care and management is carried out safely and uneventfully.

Nameband

All children should have a nameband on their wrist or ankle, correctly completed with name, date of birth and hospital number. If it needs to be removed, another should replace it immediately.

General anaesthesia

All necessary documentation must be completed, and all hospital policies carefully followed for all children who are to undergo a general anaesthetic.

Protection from infection

The hospital environment contains a variety of viruses and bacteria and, wherever possible, children need to be protected from these. Those particularly at risk are the sick, children whose natural defence systems are not efficient and the young baby whose own immune system is immature and who has yet to develop protective antibodies. Hand washing must be thorough and other necessary precautions, such as nursing the child in a cubicle, carried out.

In particular those children who are admitted to hospital as a result of an infectious disease need to be nursed in a cubicle, with both carers and family adhering to the infection control policy. This should limit the spread of infection. This subject is covered in greater detail in Chapter 6.

Drug administration

Hospital policy must be carefully followed. The child's nameband should always be checked prior to giving medicines, and no drug should ever be left unattended on tables or lockers.

Provision of sterile and correctly diluted infant feeds

Feeds, feeding equipment and dummies should be sterilized for babies up to one year of age.

Fire

All staff working within a hospital must be aware of the fire regulations and procedures.

Policies relating to all of the above points are available in your own clinical areas and you should be familiar with them. Safety is an essential component of a child's care and it is our responsibility as carers to maintain protective measures throughout the child's stay.

Protecting the child from abuse

Estimates indicate that between 150 and 200 children die each year in England and Wales from *child abuse*, and approximately 25 700 children require some protection. This is probably the tip of the iceberg and thousands more children may suffer long-term psychological problems as a result of ill treatment (Creighton & Noyes, 1989).

As you will be involved in the direct care of children – bathing, washing, talking and listening to them – it may be you who is in a position to identify either potential or actual child abuse and consequently maintain the child's safety.

What is child abuse?

There are four identified forms of abuse:

- Physical abuse
- Sexual abuse
- Neglect
- Emotional abuse

Physical abuse

'Actual or likely physical injury to a child or failure to prevent injury to a child' (Department of Health, 1992). Examples include hitting, shaking, squeezing, burning and biting the child. However, it also incorporates less immediately obvious child abuse injuries such as giving a child poisonous substances, attempted suffocation or drowning.

Neglect

'Persistent or severe neglect of a child, or failure to protect a child from exposure to any kind of danger' (Department of Health, 1992). This includes leaving children alone and unsupervised, failure to give love and attention and failure to provide for basic needs such as food, clothes, warmth and medical care.

Sexual abuse

'Actual or likely sexual exploitation of a child or adolescent' (Department of Health, 1992). This may be in the form of sexual intercourse, but also includes fondling, masturbation, oral sex, anal intercourse and exposing children to pornographic material.

Emotional abuse

'Actual or likely severe adverse effect on the emotional and behavioural development of a child caused by persistent or severe emotional ill-treatment or rejection' (Department of Health, 1992). This relates to constant lack of love and affection, threats, verbal attack, taunting and shouting, which lead to a loss of confidence and the child becomes withdrawn. All forms of abuse are likely to involve some emotional ill-treatment that is likely to have a damaging and long-lasting effect on the child.

Detecting child abuse

Abuse can have profound effects upon a child and, sadly, it is not as rare and unusual as is sometimes thought. Child abuse can affect *any* family, so prevention, early detection and supportive help and advice are crucial to the well-being of the child and family.

The most severe cases of child abuse are usually not difficult to identify, but not all incidents are clear-cut.

Activity 13.10 ■

Consider the following examples. Would you think them to be child abuse?

■ The continuation of corporal punishment in public/private schools.
■ A six-year-old girl who always has her bedtime bath with her father.
■ A mother who tells her three-year-old daughter that she is a nasty child and that no-one loves her.
■ A father who hits his eleven-year-old son with a cane when he misbehaves.
■ A 13-year-old girl who can't remember the last time that her mother cuddled or kissed her.

■ ■

There is no right or wrong answer. All situations are different. How you feel about these examples will probably depend upon your own culture, values and beliefs. This is something that we need to respect and take into account for all the families in our care. However, it is important that you are able to recognize some of the clinical signs of abuse.

Activity 13.11 ■

What factors would lead you to suspect that a child may have suffered the following types of abuse?

■ Neglect   ■ Physical abuse
■ Emotional abuse   ■ Sexual abuse

■ ■

In your notes you may have identified some of the following:

Neglect

■ The child is likely to appear unhappy and may be withdrawn or aggressive, with lingering health problems.
■ He/she may have problems at school, such as truancy.
■ The child may look unkempt, with signs of poor care, for example failure to thrive and severe nappy rash.

Physical abuse

■ There may be physical markings on the child's body, such as bruising in unusual places, scratches, bites or cigarette burns.
■ The family may have delayed reporting the incident and seeking medical attention.
■ There may be a discrepancy between the child's physical signs and the history of the incident. *For example*, an 18-month-old child with

scalds to both feet, which the parent(s) say was caused by the child stepping into a hot bath.

■ A knowledge of child development may identify that a child could not possibly have sustained the injury in the manner described. *For example*, a six-week-old baby may have bruises on the back which the parents say is the result of the baby rolling off the sofa. Babies of this age are unable to turn themselves!

■ The child or sibling(s) may have a history of previous injuries that have not been fully explained. The family may also exhibit abnormal attitudes and behaviour – they may be overprotective of the child or, conversely, they may display little interest.

Emotional abuse

■ The child is likely to appear withdrawn and nervous.
■ Personality changes may be evident and the child may have difficulty forming relationships.

Sexual abuse

■ The child may act out sexual activities in role play with a teddy or doll.
■ There may be soreness, bleeding or itchiness around the child's genital area; there may be signs of ano-genital trauma.
■ The child may display sexual knowledge beyond his/her years.
■ The child may exhibit fear towards a particular individual.
■ The child may have a low self-esteem.

From these points it will be clear that in some cases it may be difficult to identify child abuse. Perhaps one of the most important first steps in recognizing ill-treatment is to listen carefully and *believe* what the child is saying. Initial belief is especially important so that later questioning does not silence the child. Coupled with this, observation and accurate reporting of the child's activities are fundamental. The child may exhibit thoughts and feeling in drawings, poetry or play. It cannot be emphasized enough that the whole family needs to be assessed. If you are concerned that a child may have suffered abuse, discuss your worries with a senior member of staff immediately. Your response could dictate the future care and management of the child.

Caring for the child who has been abused – your own feelings

The thought of a child suffering any form of abuse may arouse very uncomfortable feelings within you. Remember that you are no different to anyone else and that it is natural for your emotions to rise. However, it is essential that you recognize these feelings and do not try to stifle them. Your own clinical area may have regular meetings or self-help groups, often facilitated by a psychologist, at which you may have the opportunity to explore your feelings. Alternatively, it may be appropriate for you to talk to one or more of your clinical colleagues who have also been involved in the child's care. Just airing your thoughts and views can help tremendously.

Although child abuse is a widespread and worrying problem, you may never encounter a child who has suffered ill-treatment. It is important to remember that by far the majority of children are loved, wanted and cared for by their families. If you do suspect child abuse do make sure that your concerns are passed on to other specialized personnel who will be able to fully investigate the situation.

Summary

We have considered some aspects of the care of children in hospital. It is of paramount importance that child and family are regarded as one in planning and providing care. A hospital visit can be potentially very traumatic for a child. However, as carers it is our responsibility to ensure that, for the majority of families, their transition from home to hospital and back home again is as smooth, safe and uneventful as possible.

Remember: A hospital stay can be a happy positive experience for child, family and carers.

References

Barrett, M. & McIntosh, M. (1982) *The Anti-social Family.* Verso, London.

Bond, J. & Bond. S. (1986) *Sociology and Health Care.* Churchill Livingstone, Edinburgh.

Bowlby, J. (1951) *Maternal Care and Mental Health.* World Health Organization, Geneva.

Bowlby, J. (1969) *Attachment and Loss: Volume 1 Attachment.* Hogarth Press, London.

Clark, M.H. (1987) *Where are the Children?* Caring for Children in the Health Services. Collins, London.

Child Accident Prevention Trust (1989) *Basic Principles of Child Accident Prevention: A Guide to Action.* Child Accident Prevention Trust, London.

Creighton, S.J. & Noyes, P. (1989) *Child Abuse Trends in England and Wales 1983–1987.* NSPCC, London.

Department of Health (1992) *Child Protection: Guidance for Senior Nurses, Health Visitors and Midwives.* HMSO, London.

Levene, S. & Bonfield, G. (1991) Accidents on hospital wards. *Archives of Disease in Childhood,* **66,** 1047–9.

Ministry of Health (1959) *The Welfare of Children in Hospital. Report of the Committee.* HMSO, London.

Murdock, G.P. (1965) *Social Structure.* The Free Press USA (Purnell Distribution Centre, Bristol).

National Voluntary Council for Children's Play (1992) *The Charter for Children's Play.* Children's Society, London.

Play in Hospital Liaison Committee (1990) *Quality Management for Children. Play in Hospital.* Play in Hospital Liaison Committee, London.

Robertson, J. (1958) *Young Children in Hospital.* Tavistock Publications, London.

Shannon, F.T., Ferguson, D.M. & Dimond, M.E. (1984) Early hospital admissions and subsequent behavioural problems in 6 year olds. *Archives of Disease in Childhood*, **59**, 815–19.

Worsley, P. (Ed) (1977) *Introducing Sociology*, 2nd edn. Penguin Books, Harmondsworth.

Further reading

Baxter, C. (1989) Race and child abuse. *Health Visitor*, September, **62**, 271–2.

Clark, M.C.M. (1989) In what ways, if any, are child abusers different from other parents? *Health Visitor*, September, **62**, 268–70.

Department of Health (1991) *Welfare of Children and Young People in Hospital.* HMSO, London.

Eiser, C. & Hanson, L. (1989) Preparing children for hospital: a school-based intervention. *Professional Nurse*, March, **4**(6), 297–300.

Fradd, E. (1986) Learning about hospital. *Nursing Times*, 15 January, **82**(3), 28–30.

Frost, N. & Stein, N. (1989) *The Politics of Child Welfare.* Harvester Wheatsheaf, London.

Goodman, S. & Adams, C. (1989) "Uncumphatable". *Nursing Times*, 6 December, **85**(49), 28–31.

Hall, D. & Stacey, M. (Eds) (1979) *Beyond Separation.* Routledge & Kegan Paul, London.

Hawthorn, P. (1974) *Nurse – I Want my Mummy!* Royal College of Nursing, London.

Jessel, C. (1990) *Birth to Three: Parents' Guide to Child Development.* Bloomsbury Publishing, London.

Matterson, E. (1989) *Play with a Purpose*, 3rd edn. Penguin Books, Harmondsworth.

Meehan, F. (1991) Suffer the little children. *Nursing*, 24 January–13 February, **4**(27), 16–17.

Petrillo, M. & Sanger, S. (1980) *Emotional Care of Hospitalised Children*, 2nd edn. J.B. Lippincott, Philadelphia.

Rutter, M. (1972) *Maternal Deprivation Reassessed.* Penguin Books, Harmondsworth.

Save the Children (1989) *Hospital: A Deprived Environment for Children? The Case for Hospital Playschemes.* Save the Children, London.

Weller, B.F. (1980) *Helping Sick Children to Play.* Balliere Tindall, London.

Webborn, J. & Laryea, P. (1991) Acts of power. *Nursing*, 24 January–13 February, **4**(27), 14–15.

West, J. (1992) *Child-centred Play Therapy.* Edward Arnold, London.

Books to aid a child's preparation for hospitalization and medical procedures

Adamson, J. & Adamson G. (1988) *Topsy and Tim go to Hospital.* Blackie and Son, London.

Bawden, J. (1989) *When I went to Hospital.* Little Mammoth, London.
NAWCH (1980) *Andrew goes for an X-Ray.* National Association for the Welfare of Children in Hospital, London.
Taylor Cork, B. (1989) *Going to the Hospital.* Conran Octopus, London.
Wade, B. (1981) *Linda goes to Hospital.* A & C Black, London.
Wells. P. (1985) *Talkabout going into Hospital.* Ladybird, London.

Chapter 14
Community Care
Joan Harding

Overview

This chapter examines community care. It helps to identify circumstances in which care is given outside institutions/hospitals and make some comparisons between the two. It also explores the special relationships between carers and clients. It describes the organization of community care and the care team.

Key words

Individual, home, rights, privacy, guests/visitors, property, support, care team.

The community

Care in the community is usually taken to mean care in the *home* of the *individual* client. Traditionally the principal groups cared for have been the elderly, individuals with learning disabilities (mental handicap) and those of all ages with physical disabilities.

But what do we mean exactly by the term *community*? It means different things to different people, but for our purpose we might consider:

- The place
- The activity
- The people
- Understanding

Care at home therefore must take into account the client, the situation, the family and the community in which the client lives.

Activity 14.1 ■

 Consider your own community and especially those features which influence your daily life. How comprehensive are they? Consider if you were to be discharged from hospital and were to need *local support systems*, what connections would you need? Do you have them?

■ ■

By now your views of the community may be changing. This then is the kind of background situation against or amid which community (sometimes called domiciliary) care is given.

Differences between care at home and in hospital

Care in the client's home does mean being able to adapt well learned principles of care to the particular setting of home, especially where facilities may not be like those of a hospital or residential home and indeed may not be the same as those we are used to in our own homes. However, this is where the client lives, where their roots and own belongings are.

Activity 14.2 ■■■■■■■■■■■■■■■■■■■■■■■■■■■

 Try to identify some of the differences between care at home and in hospital.

■■■■■■■■■■■■■■■■■■■■■■■■■■■■■■■■

Your list might include some of the following:

- ■ Participation in care
- ■ Individual *rights*
- ■ Client expectations
- ■ Illness/health orientation
- ■ Who is in charge/has the power

- ■ Exercise of choice
- ■ Individual identity
- ■ Uniform and status
- ■ Short–long-term care

Looking at these differences it is clear that community care is more likely to be a longer-term undertaking, and therefore the relationship between client and carer(s) becomes a special one which develops with time. Indeed such relationships often become lifetime friendships, not only with the client but with the family too.

It is important to remember that carers in the client's home are *visitors* or *guests* and that although close relationships are often established, this guest status does not change. Carers therefore must always be mindful of their position.

Recipients of community care

Did you know?

Ninety per cent of health care delivered to clients is given in the community. This does include clinics and surgeries, but the greater part is given at home. Only 5% of people aged 65 or over needing care are in an institution. The remainder are in their own homes looking after themselves or being cared for by relatives, friends or community nurses.

Clients who are acutely ill, of course, also receive care at home, more usually on a short-term basis anticipating complete recovery. This group is likely to increase in size with the changing pattern of hospital care and the trends toward short stay and early discharge, which often means continuing or completing care at home. This growing activity emphasizes the need for careful discharge planning and community carers are now called upon to provide an *ever* widening range of care, calling for more skills and a larger work force or team.

Finally, the care group comprises a growing number of people who are not ill but who need assistance to enable them to lead their daily lives in their own homes, therefore increasing the demand for services and carers.

Referrals for community care

Activity 14.3 ■

 Take a few minutes to think in detail about where referrals for care in the community may come from.

■ ■

Does your list include:

- Antenatal clinics?
- General practitioners?
- Hospitals (liaison)?
- Social Services and other local authority departments, e.g. Housing?
- Neighbours and friends?
- Old people's homes, nursing homes, residential homes?

- New births?
- Self-referral?
- Teachers, education and welfare officers?
- Relatives?
- Voluntary agencies?
- The police?

Your list is probably even more extensive, ample evidence of the very diverse range of settings in which care may be given.

Services required in community care

This leads us on to consider the range of care that may be required:

- The client may need general care, assistance with personal hygiene and grooming.

- The need may be for promotion of living skills, mobility and rehabilitation.
- The client may need assistance with eating and drinking, or need to be fed via a nasogastric tube.
- The client may have returned from a hospital admission and need assistance or follow up to care started in hospital, for example, dressings, stoma care or special treatments.
- Finally the client may need advice and teaching for health promotion. This kind of care would be particularly relevant for mothers with children (Fig. 14.1) or for clients who have undergone some dramatic change in their health status, for example following a heart attack or stroke.

Activity 14.4   ■

Think of some clients with whose care you have been involved and write a few lines to remind yourself of all the items of care they needed and were given. If you were to exchange notes with a colleague at this stage you are likely to find that each of you describes a completely different set of circumstances.

■ ■

This pinpoints three further issues to consider:

(1)   The importance of liaison in referring clients for care at home
(2)   The growing range of client groups who need this care
(3)   The organization of care in the community

Fig. 14.1 Mother and baby attending a health centre.

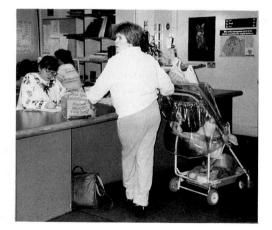

Liaison in client referral

Successful liaison relies on the effective gathering, recording and transmission of details about a client's care so that it can continue without interruption or omissions. In many instances liaison nurses and health visitors visit hospital wards, clinics and departments to gather information about clients who need follow-up care. In some cases these activities play a crucial part in preparing to receive clients home and continue their care uninterrupted.

Client groups needing care

Earlier in this chapter reference was made to possible client groups who have made up the majority receiving community health care. After completing Activity 14.3 it will have become clear that this range is much wider and includes:

- Mothers and babies
- Adults
- The handicapped
- Those who have suffered injury/trauma
- The mentally ill

- Children
- The elderly
- The acutely or temporarily ill
- The long-term sick, young or old
- The dying

The care needs of such diverse client groups are bound to have similarities and differences and no one group of carers could be expected to have all the skills needed for delivering care. Therefore we see different carers developing expertise in the care of certain groups and the subsequent emergence of *care teams*.

Organization of care

The term with which we should all be familiar in describing community care is *primary health care*. We should also be certain that we understand what it means. A working definition was given by the World Health Organization (1978):

Primary health care is essential health care made universally accessible to individuals and families in the community by means acceptable to them through their full participation and at a cost that the community and country can afford. It forms an integral part of the country's health system of which it is the main focus.

It is the first level of contact of individuals, the family and the community with the national health system, bringing health care as close as possible to where people live and work.

Primary health care team

The primary health care team in the broadest sense includes all agencies whose function is to provide primary care. Figure 14.2 illustrates a health centre, displaying health promotion information. In considering the smaller team of nurses/carers meeting the needs of the clients we have already identified the team as consisting of:

- District nurses
- Health visitors
- Practice nurses
- School nurses
- Occupational health nurses
- Community midwives
- Community psychiatric nurses
- Community mental handicap nurses
- Specialist nurses:
    Diabetic liaison
    Incontinence advisor
    Family planning nurse

Activity 14.5 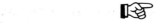 ■

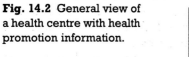 As a care assistant you may find yourself reporting to any of these professionals in the course of your work so it would be sensible to make the effort to have some understanding of their various *roles* in health care. You might also make contact with nurses in your area and hear from them about their day-to-day work.

■ ■

Fig. 14.2 General view of a health centre with health promotion information.

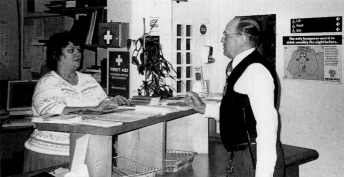

Nature of community care

Workloads vary according to the characteristics of the locality, for example a large elderly population, travelling families, bed and breakfast accommodation, young families with small children, under fives and school age children, ethnic populations. The community care service, therefore, needs to be flexible to meet demand.

In considering the details of care given to clients in the community many of the principles and procedures discussed in the earlier chapters of this book will apply, adapted to suit the individual client and the particular home circumstances.

Areas of special care are increasing, especially the care of the elderly, care of clients with learning difficulties (mental handicap) and care of the dying. More people are choosing to die at home among their families and loved ones. This has led to the growth of *special support teams*. Many people are aware of these now, and also of the work undertaken by Macmillan nurses and others with special skills. The main aims of such teams are to respond to individual needs to give care and support to the client and their family.

Six million people are cared for at home by relatives. This does represent an enormous burden which persists for some for 24 hours each day, seven days each week and for each week of the year. The greater part of this burden is taken by women, sometimes with little awareness of help that could be available.

Assessment of the needs of carers is basically an extension to assessment of the client's needs. Remember that the well-being of the family is of equal importance to that of the client. Their needs can be wide ranging: some purely practical, for example a hoist to help lift and move an increasingly handicapped client, or more complex, focusing on the emotional and psychological effects of caring. Some examples of the second category are:

- The loss experienced in watching the physical and mental deterioration of a loved one, for example one partner with senile dementia who is 'No longer the person I married'.
- The mentally handicapped child who grows physically but whose mental development does not keep pace – a child in an adult body.
- The guilt and resentment arising from feeling caught by the circumstances of incapacity or financial constraints.
- The seemingly interminable burden on the carer's shoulders with lack of time to themselves for refreshment or leisure.
- The stress of caring when the previous relationship was not a very good one, for example when an only daughter who did not get on very well with her mother becomes her sole carer in later life.
- The inability to express one's feelings leads to an emotionally taxing charade.

In such circumstances the notion of *respite care* – knowing that somebody else will care for one weekend a month or that the patient can go for a fortnight's stay in a hospice, elderly unit or child nursery – will make all the difference. The need for these services must be identified and forward planning is necessary, as there is no doubt of the benefit to all concerned.

National Health Service and Community Care Act 1990

As demands for care in the community increase so does the need to organize its provision. The chief recommendations of the Griffiths Report (1988), undertaken to identify these needs, were that local authority social service departments should be responsible for identifying people with community care needs in an area and negotiating with other agencies. This would mean an interactive planning relationship between social services, health authorities and other service-providing agencies.

The Government white paper, Community Care in the Next Decade and Beyond, (1989) reinforced the belief that for most people well organized community care offers the best form of care available. The intention expressed in the white paper is to help people to lead, as far as possible, independent lives in their own homes, provided with the right amount of support and care, and to give them a greater individual say in how they live their lives and in what services they need to help them do so.

The six key objectives for service delivery in the community area:

- To promote the development of domiciliary, day and respite services to enable people to live in their own homes wherever feasible and sensible.
- To ensure that service providers make practical support for carers a high priority.
- To make proper assessment of need and good case management the corner stone of high quality care.
- To promote the development of a flourishing independent sector alongside good quality public services.
- To clarify the responsibilities of agencies and so make it easier to hold them to account for their performance.
- To secure better value for taxpayers' money by introducing a new funding structure for social care.

The Act has become law and is being implemented. Carers will witness and be involved in changes as new arrangements are introduced covering individual care to the full range of clients in the community whom we identified earlier in this chapter.

Summary

The nature of care in the community is very diverse and the client needing care at *home* may require help with many aspects of daily living to enable them to achieve physical, social and emotional well-being. Families may undertake many of these tasks, but still rely on health workers to provide services and *support* or, at times, take on the activities completely.

Care must be based on an appreciation of *individual* needs and it must be given in a sensitive and thoughtful way. The carer must take into account their own *visitor* status in the client's home and also acknowledge the client's *rights* to:

- Enjoy as normal a life as possible within the community
- Receive health care to facilitate this normal life
- Be treated as an individual among their own property and possessions

References

Luker, K., O. & J. (Eds) (1985) *Health Visiting.* Blackwell Scientific Publications, Oxford.

WHO (1978) *Primary Health Care: Report of the International Conference on Primary Health Care, Asta, USSR.* WHO, Geneva.

Community Care: Agenda for Action (Griffiths Report, April 1988). HMSO, London.

Caring for People. Community Care in the Next Decade and Beyond. (November, 1989). HMSO, London.

Further reading

Baker, G., Bevan, J.M. McDonnell & Wall, B. (1987) *Community Nursing: Research 4, Recent Developments.* Croom Helm, London.

McMurray, A. (1990) *Community Health Nursing – Primary Health Care in Practice.* Churchill Livingstone, Edinburgh.

Meredith-Davies, B. (1991) *Community Health and Social Services*, 5th edn. Edward Arnold, Sevenoaks.

Ottewell, R.P. & Wall, A. (1990) *The Growth and Development of the Community Health Services.* Business Educational Publishers, Sunderland.

Chapter 15
Caring for the Patient and Their Family Facing Loss
Elizabeth Atchison

Overview

In this chapter we will consider the care of the person facing death and loss. The psychological, spiritual, religious and social support will be taken into account. In addition we will look at the needs of the carer and ourselves, as only by learning about ourselves can we also learn to care for others, in particular as we face this difficult but most important stage of life. Different aspects of the support that might be given to patients and their families are illustrated in Fig. 15.1.

The term *patient* is used throughout the chapter as this more accurately sets the relationship between the *cared for* and the carer. The physical care of the patient who is dying will not be covered in detail. Refer back to other chapters in this book for specific help concerning, for example, hygiene, comfort and rest and other areas of care. We must not forget that the dying patient may need the maximum amount of care.

Key words

Loss, grief, grieving, bereavement, spiritual, culture, religion, dignity.

Loss

The experience of *losing* something is one which we encounter frequently throughout life. Bowlby (1969, 1973, 1980) talks of loss, separation and

Fig. 15.1 Dimensions of support for clients and their families.

Physical support	Psychological support
Spiritual and religious support	Social support

detachment. Many other writers also include the experience of loss as being most important in our development.

If we think back to our first losses they would include perhaps, birth itself, mother going off to work or losing a toy. The quality of this experience and the support we receive during it goes with us and guides the way we cope in adult life.

Activity 15.1 ■

Think about an *item* you have lost recently, for example a train ticket. Note down some of the feelings you had and perhaps what you did.

■ ■

In your notes you may have recorded some of the following things:

Feelings

Sad, anxious, panic, disbelief, cross or angry, lonely, frightened, shocked.

Actions

Searching, contacting someone who could help, going back to the place where it occurred, trying to recollect your last steps. Later on you may have told several people about this experience and how you felt.

Some losses are obviously more important than others. This guides the intensity of the feelings we describe above. The greater the experience of loss, the more painful. Also the greater the loss, the longer the time needed to recover. The loss does not have to be valuable in the sense of money, it depends rather on how important it is to us. For example, if we lost a plastic ring it would be cheap to replace, but if it was given to us by a childhood friend it may be very symbolic and be a real treasure that money could not replace.

What makes some losses more difficult than others?

The feelings of loss are a unique experience. Nobody ever feels exactly the same although, as we have just discovered, there is some common ground. Many variables make some losses more difficult:

(1) The persons we are. As unique individuals our previous experience of loss, the way we coped and the support available play a part.
(2) The circumstances in which the loss occurs, and our ability to make sense of it.
(3) To some extent, the time scale. If we know we are moving house, we can prepare for it. We have time to think about what it would be like not to live there; time to go round and see or do all the favourite things for the last time. If, however, the house is burnt down suddenly,

accepting that the house will no longer be there and that we will no longer be able to do all these favourite things will perhaps make the loss more difficult. Whether the house is fairly new to us or a long-standing family home will also change the significance of the loss.

How does this knowledge of loss help us to care for patients?

When we are supporting patients and their families they may be experiencing many losses at once. Each loss will have its own significance.

Activity 15.2 ■

 List some of the many losses a seriously ill or dying patient or their family may go through.

■ ■

You may have come up with some of the following ideas or many more!

Patient

Health, mobility, independence, weight, financial income, youth, dignity, role, faith.

Family

Home, financial income, a family member, security, hope, company.

Human beings need to establish bonds with people and objects. As life goes on these bonds are strengthened and broken as part of life's rich tapestry. From what we have said so far life would seem less painful if we did not take people and things to our hearts. Yet how lonely life would be in isolation – not giving or receiving love and affection. As was once said 'only whose who know love can experience grief'. The two are intertwined. Few would choose not to share the richness of loving.

Grief, grieving and bereavement

The death of a loved one brings with it the greatest challenge to our whole existence. Perhaps it is the greatest *loss*. Some would say that the losses we experience in earlier life are our preparation, but this can only be true if we know how to learn from them.

Activity 15.3 ■

 Think about the loss you described in Activity 15.1. Consider what you would do differently and what would have made you feel better.

■ ■

The word *grief* is often used to describe multiple feelings and emotions of deep sorrow associated with loss. *Grieving* is the state of feeling grief and *bereavement* is the time span or episode during which this occurs. Many authors have described the emotions of grieving and the feelings of grief. They have done this through years of working with people who are facing death or who have lost a loved one. This does not reduce the uniqueness of the individual's responses, but helps us to see the common ground, so that as carers we can try to understand and support patients.

Anticipatory grief

The most commonly recognized person to be experiencing grief is the person left behind, but there are two important additional times when people may be grieving:

(1)   If the relative *knows* in advance that their loved one is going to die, they may start their grieving process *before* the actual death occurs – grieving in anticipation, we could say.
(2)   When the patient is facing their own death. This grief may be due to many losses: the loss of their own life; leaving their loved ones behind; the dreams, hopes and expectations that may be unfulfilled.

Activity 15.4   ■

Make a list of all the people who might grieve following the death of a patient.

■ ■

In fact, anybody who knows your patient may be affected to some degree and that includes us, the carers. Some of those who may be affected by the grief following the death of a patient are identified in Fig. 15.2.

Tasks of mourning to work through

This section is based on the work of William Worden (1991) who wrote about the tasks of mourning (mourning and grieving being the same) that those suffering a loss might work through. Looking at these tasks may help guide us as carers, particularly in the support we may offer our patients and their families.

When people experience the loss of a loved one, to get back to a time when life again seems normal appears impossible. However, through the process of *grief work* and by completing the *tasks of mourning* life can again become bearable. It is important to remember that grief work is a process of moving forward and not going back to how things were. Part of the help a carer or supporter can give at this time is to be there and to listen.

For those experiencing grief the future is often like looking through a

Fig. 15.2 Those who may be affected by grief following the death of a patient.

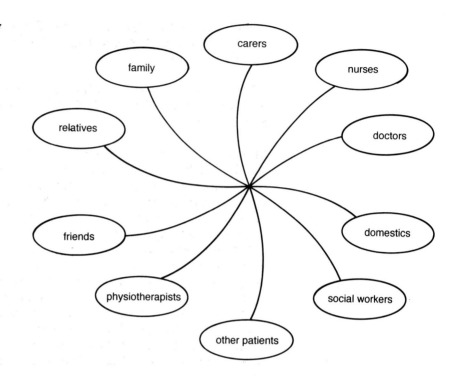

closed door. It is impossible to imagine at that time. The journey is slow and hindered by a longing for the past which at times appears unmanageable. But the future can be bright for those who have experienced grief; it can become a time when memories of the past and the picture of the future can live comfortably side by side.

We will cover the tasks of mourning, as identified by Worden (1991), in some detail.

Task 1: to accept the reality of the loss

As already mentioned, accepting that something has actually happened is one of the first thoughts and emotions to grapple with in dealing with loss. We may hear people say:

> It can't be true
> It can't be me
> The report must be wrong
> The notes must be muddled.

Before anything else this reality has to be faced. It is however a process, not a one-off event. Therefore patients and their families may need to be given the opportunity to ask questions, again and again, phrasing their requests in different ways. The role of the carer is to listen and be around. Senior staff should be involved if the patient or family are asking for more information than the carer is able to give. Comfort should be offered where necessary. It is important to note that this task is handled in the patient's own time and pace.

The family who have recently had a loved one die may need to return to the ward or place of death to check their loved one is not there. This is a kind of searching process.

Task 2: to work through the pain of grief

Worden feels it is impossible to lose a loved one without feeling some pain. Again, this is an individual experience. However, we cannot escape this emotional pain; if it is ignored it may only be postponed and may emerge much later. People may show their pain in many ways; anger, depression, sadness, anxiety and fear are examples.

The carer can do much by just being with people during this difficult time as often people do not want to be alone. It is important to remember that the pain is due to the loss, not the carer's presence. When somebody is telling their story and cries, it is the pain of loss not the telling us that hurts.

People may find that they are avoided by their friends and supporters. This is often because people don't know what to say. We must not fall into the same trap. Just being there is often a great comfort. Be honest, say 'I don't know what to say'. This is often better than saying the wrong thing, but thoughtful silence is just as helpful.

Task 3: to adjust to an environment in which the deceased is missing

After the loss of a loved one this task is concerned with the practical issues as well as the emotional ones. For those anticipating the loss, this time is like a role reversal where they can think through how they might manage. Jarvis (1958) called this 'worry work'. It is an important part of the grieving process.

It is not helped by carers saying 'don't worry, it will all work out', as worry work is an intricate part of the process of adjustment. However, the support of the carer is again crucial. Perhaps it would be helpful to talk through financial and social problems with other members of the multi-disciplinary team, for example the social worker. The carer can notify a member of senior staff who will contact them.

Task 4: to find a safe place for the deceased in their emotions and move on with life

The final task brings us back to the beginning of this discussion, where the future and the past can walk comfortably hand in hand. Nobody forgets and nobody goes back to the past either. Perhaps at the time of reconciliation a new type of person emerges or a new stage in life commences.

How do we know when grieving has finished? We know this when the periods between the pain become longer, when the future can again be planned for, when life is bearable again. This does not mean that the loved one is forgotten. The changes made in the grieving person's life go on in their thoughts, actions, dreams and memories. A time arrives when special occasions come round and these periods of remembering are with a smile, rather than tears.

Activity 15.5 ■

 When you are next caring for a dying patient and their family, think about Task 1 and make some notes on how both the patient and the family begin to accept the reality of the situation.

■ ■

Spiritual care

Everybody may have a *spiritual* aspect. Some people call it their soul, others the inner energy that makes them who they are. Often *spirituality* is linked with *religious* beliefs and followings, but for those without religious beliefs questions such as: 'Who am I?', 'What has been the purpose of my life?', 'What does the end mean?' are a complex part of their spiritual make-up. Often these questions are unanswerable. In fact one answer will not be right for all, as the answers need to be as individual as the people who are asking and perhaps can only be answered by themselves.

Facing death is a vulnerable and sensitive time. Patients ask questions not knowing or wanting an answer. Or perhaps they may ask 'what do you believe?'. The sharing of our beliefs when asked helps patients to form a picture, perhaps to accept, reject or explore further the need for their own answers. For just as clients are individual, so are the members of the caring team. It is this mixture of people and their beliefs which makes life so rich. However, we should be careful not to offer our beliefs when they are not called or asked for.

Spirituality was once described as a candle flame burning brightly inside (Fig. 15.3). We can feed the flame by allowing patients to be free to choose what is right for them. Giving freedom of choice and respecting individuality may help the patient find their own way.

Religious and cultural beliefs

Our *culture* is learned from the place and group we predominantly grow up in. It is made of values, beliefs, attitudes and social awareness (refer to Chapter 1 concerning the individuality of the client). However, people brought up in the same area may have different religious and cultural beliefs. Often religion and culture are inseparable and the understanding of people's wishes is therefore complex. In this section we will look at the need of certain religious groups, not forgetting that these are broad

Fig. 15.3 Candle.

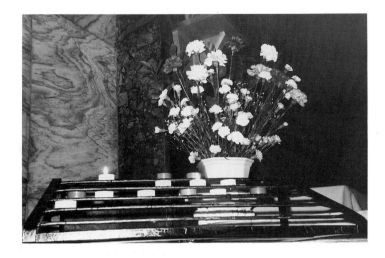

guidelines. For example the patient who says they are Christian may have a variable degree of commitment to this belief. This may also be true for those holding any of the other religious beliefs. The only way to be sure and not to offend is to ask.

The following outline is very brief and contains only the special needs concerned with the time of death.

Muslim patients

At the time of death

The patient may wish to face Mecca. Prayers may be recited by the family.

Handling of the body

After the death the patient's body should not be touched by non-Muslims. If this is unavoidable the carer should wear disposable gloves.

After death

Muslims are always buried.

Sikh patients

At the time of death

The patient may receive comfort from reciting from their holy book.

Handling of the body

Non-Sikh carers may touch the body. Families will wish to be involved in last ceremonies. Some Sikhs take an extra vow and abide by the five articles. They wear a wrist band, a short sword, a wooden comb, cotton shorts and do not cut their hair, which is covered by a turban for male Sikhs. These articles should not be touched or removed, nor the hair cut.

After death

Sikhs are always cremated. This should take place as soon as possible.

Jewish patients

There is a wide spectrum of observance amongst Jewish patients and carers should always check their wishes. Jewish patients hold the preservation of life as very important.

At the time of death

The patient may wish to recite prayers with the family.

Handling of the body

The body should be touched as little as possible.

After death

Jews are usually buried. Jewish people have a burial society in the community which handles all the preparations.

Hindu patients

At the time of death

The patient may receive comfort from hymns and readings. The Hindu priest may perform holy rites. If at all possible, the patient will wish to be at home.

Handling of the body

The body should not be touched by non-Hindus and disposable gloves should be worn if necessary. Do not remove jewellery or sacred threads from the body.

After the death

All adult Hindus are cremated.

Buddhist patients

At the time of death

The Buddhist may wish to have peace and quiet. The relaxed state of mind is very important. Chanting may be used by fellow Buddhists to help this.

Handling of the body

Normal practice may be followed. Contact a Buddhist monk.

After death

Most Buddhists prefer cremation and then the ashes are buried.

Christian patients

At the time of death

The patient may wish to recite prayers. The priest may be called to perform blessing of the sick.

Handling of the body

Normal hospital practice.

After death

Burial or cremation is often a personal preference.

This section is only a guide and does not replace the importance of establishing individual wishes of the patient and the family.

Activity 15.6 ■

 Find out who is the link person in the community for the above religious groups and how they may be contacted.

■ ■

Maintaining dignity

After somebody dies it is the responsibility of the carer to maintain the *dignity* of that person, both for them and the family who leave them in our care and safe keeping. Not forgetting the above religious preferences, the family themselves may wish to be involved in the last care, often called the *last offices*. The care itself may vary slightly, but what is offered here is an overall guide.

Last offices

Following death of the patient, the doctor who has been caring for them during the last illness is required to confirm the death and issue a certificate. Once this has occurred, the carer will straighten the body and lie the patient flat. Eyelids and mouth should be closed, supporting the jaw with a pillow if necessary. Now the procedure normally used in caring for the patient's hygiene needs is performed: washing, shaving, cleaning nails and combing and arranging hair. Any equipment still attached to the patient is normally removed, unless there are special circumstances.

The body is then dressed in a shroud. Check that identity bracelets are present, both at the wrist and ankle. Also it is usual to complete two notification of death cards, one of which is taped on to the shroud. Finally the body is placed in a body bag and secured. The second card is secured to the bag top. Practices may vary from place to place, but procedures should be conducted in a quiet and respectful way.

Activity 15.7 ■

 At your place of work look for the procedure book and read the section on last offices. Note any special instructions which apply.

Activity 15.8 ■

 If your loved one died in hospital, a home or hospice how would you prefer their dignity to be maintained? You may like to share this activity with a colleague(s) and discuss it together.

■ ■

Caring for the carer

The material in this chapter covers delicate and sensitive issues. When we care for patients and their families it reminds us that we are mortal too and will one day die. It may also bring reminders and feelings of our own losses, or perhaps by caring for a man who looks like our own father we realize that our father won't be around for ever.

In addition to this we too face a grieving process, and have an adaptation to loss to make when the patient for whom we have been caring dies. Often we have built a very special bond and may have learned much from the way in which they faced death.

Summary

We have reviewed the areas of loss, grief and bereavement and identified some principles for dealing with these situations. We must not forget that grief is a normal and necessary response to loss. For the patient and their family the support they receive from carers is vital. As carers we are in the privileged position to help patients and families to start their long journey through loss in a positive and supportive way.

References

Bowlby, J. (1969) *Attachment*. Basic Books, New York.

Bowlby, J. (1973) *Separation*. Basic Books, New York.

Bowlby, J. (1980) *Loss*. Basic Books, New York.

Janis, J. (1958) *Psychological Distress, Psychoanalytical and Behavioural Studies of Surgical Patients*. Chapman and Hall, London.

Worden, J.W. (1991) *Grief Counselling and Grief Therapy. A Handbook for the Mental Health Practitioner*, 2nd edn. Tavistock, London.

Further reading

Canis, P. (1992) Attending the spirit. *Nursing Times*, 5 August, **88**(32), 50.

Copperman, H. (1983) *Dying at Home*. Pitman Press, Bath.

Gorer, G. (1980) *Death, Grief and Mourning in Contemporary Britain*. Crescent Press, London.

Green, J. (1992) *Death with dignity, meeting the spiritual needs of patients in a multi-cultural society*. Macmillan, Basingstoke.

Green, J. (1992) Death with dignity. *Nursing Times*, 15 January, **88**(3), 25–9.

Kershaw, B., Wright, S. & Hammonds, P. (1980) *Helping to Care – a Handbook for Carers at Home and in Hospital*, Chapter 14. Bailliere Tindall, London.

Kubler-Ross, E. (1970) *On Death and Dying*. Tavistock Routledge, London.

Lugton, J. (1987) *Communication with Dying People and their Relatives*. Lisa Sainsbury Foundation. Austen Cornish, London.

McGilloway, D. (1988) *Nursing and Spiritual Care*. Harper Row, London.

Morrison, R. (1992) Diagnosing spiritual pain in patients. *Nursing Standard*, 11 March, **6**(25), 36–8.

Neuberger, J. (1987) Caring for dying people of different faiths. Lisa Sainsbury Foundation. Austin Cornish, London.

Parkes, C.M. (1986) *Bereavement: Studies of Grief in Adult Life*, 2nd edn. Tavistock, London.

Riggans, L. (1992) Living with loss. *Nursing Times*, 1 July, **88**(27), 34–5.

Sadler, C. (1992) A good death. *Nursing Times*, 29 July, **88**(31), 16–17.

Wiseman, C. (1992) Bereavement care in an acute ward. *Nursing Times*, 13 May, **88**(2), 34–5.

Cross-reference with NVQ/SVQ

Christine McMahon

This appendix cross-references the contents of the book with some of the units of competence as they appear in the National Occupational Standards for the Care NVQ at levels 2 and 3. This book does not cover all of the 20 available awards for an NVQ in Care. It does however contain some of the underpinning knowledge required for the core units, for both levels 2 and 3; this is to be found in Section 1 of the book.

Section 2 of this book covers the level 2 Care Award: Direct Care and some of these units are to be found in other endorsements.

Section 3 of this book contains the underpinning knowledge for the level 2 Care Award covering the Postnatal Care endorsement and the level 3 Care Award covering the following endorsements: Acute Care, Adults and Acute Care, Young Children. Some of the units for the level 3 endorsements, including Terminal Care: Clinic and Outpatient care, can also be found in this section.

As each chapter is not a definitive work, further reading has been included at the end of each. It should be possible to locate the appropriate journals and books in any library within a College of Nursing or possibly in your local public library.

Unit of competence/element	Chapter
0 unit Promote equality for all individuals This is to be found in all chapters, but primarily in the following:	
(a) Promote anti-discriminatory practice.	1, 7, 8, 9, 12, 13, 15
(b) Maintain confidentiality of information.	1, 4
(c) Promote and support individual rights and choice within service delivery.	1, 7, 8, 9, 12, 13, 15
(d) Acknowledge individuals' personal beliefs and identity.	1, 7, 8, 9, 12, 13, 15
(e) Support individuals through effective communication.	2, 3
Z1 unit Contribute to the protection of individuals from abuse	
(b) Minimize the negative effects of disruptive or abusive behaviour.	3, 13

Unit of competence/element	Chapter

Z3 unit Contribute to the management of aggressive and abusive behaviour

(a) Contribute to the promotion of non-aggressive and non-abusive behaviour. — 3

(b) Contribute to the management of episodes of aggressive or abusive behaviour to clients. — 3

Z4 unit Promote communication with the client where there are communication difficulties

(a) Obtain and agree information on client communication abilities. — 2

(b) Assist client to communicate. — 2

Z7 unit Contribute to the movement and treatment of clients to maximise their physical comfort

(a) Prepare the client and environment for moving and lifting. — 5

(b) Assist the client to move from one position to another. — 5

(c) Assist the client to prevent and minimize adverse effects of pressure. — 10

Z9 unit Enable the clients to maintain their personal hygiene and appearance.

(a) Enable the clients to maintain personal cleanliness. — 8

(b) Support clients in personal grooming and dressing. — 8

Z10 unit Enable the clients to eat and drink

(a) Enable the clients to choose appropriate food and drink. — 9

(b) Enable the clients to prepare for eating and drinking. — 9, 6

(c) Assist the clients with eating and drinking. — 9, 6

Z11 unit Enable the client to access and use toilet facilities

(a) Enable the clients to access toilet facilities. — 7

(b) Assist clients to use toilet facilities. — 7

(c) Collect and dispose of clients' body waste. — 7, 6

Z14 unit Support clients and others at times of loss

(a) Support clients, their partners, relatives and friends in their initial adjustment to learning of the client during loss or death. — 15

(b) Support clients during loss or death. — 15

(c) Comfort and support the partner, relatives and friends of those who have died or suffered a loss. — 15

Unit of competence/element	Chapter

Z15 unit Contribute to care of a deceased person
(a) Assist in the preparation of a deceased person   15
    prior to the removal from the care environment.

Z16 unit Care for the baby in the first ten days of life
(a) Care for the baby's hygiene and well-being   12
    during the first ten days of life.
(b) Feed and interact with the baby.   12

Z19 unit Enable clients to achieve physical comfort
(a) Assist in minimizing discomfort and pain.   10
(b) Assist in providing conditions to meet clients'   10
    need for rest.

Z20 unit Care for and promote the development of babies in the first year of their lives
(a) Fulfil the nutritional needs of the baby.   13
(b) Manage the physical care of babies.   13
(b) Promote the physical growth and development   13
    of babies.
(d) Provide stimulation to foster the development of 13
    babies.
(e) Promote the language development of babies.   13

X12 unit Support the professionals with clinical activities
(a) Prepare the clients for treatment, investigation 11
    or procedures.
(b) Support clients and professionals during   11
    treatment, investigations or procedures.
(c) Assist the clients to recover from treatments,   11
    investigations or procedures.

X13 unit Prepare and undertake agreed clinical activities with clients whose health is stable in non-acute settings
(a) Prepare clients for clinical activities.   11, 13
(c) Obtain specimens from clients.   11, 13

X19 unit Prepare and undertake agreed on-going clinical activities with clients in acute care settings
(a) Prepare clients for clinical activities.   11, 13
(c) Obtain specimens.   11, 13

W1 unit Support clients in developing their identity and personal relationships
(d) Support clients' expressions of sexuality and   1
    sexual activity.

Unit of competence/element	Chapter

*W6 unit Reinforce professional advice through
supporting and encouraging the mothers in active
parenting in the first days of babies' lives*

(a) Assist mothers to care for babies' safety, protection and security.	12
(b) Assist mothers in caring for babies' hygiene and well-being.	12
(c) Support mothers in feeding babies.	12

*W7 unit Support and encourage parents and others
to care for babies during the first year of their life*

(a) Enable parents and others to care for babies' safety, protection and security.	13
(b) Enable parents and others to care for babies' hygiene and well-being.	13
(c) Enable parents and others to feed babies.	13

*U3 unit Prepare and maintain environments for
clinical procedures*

(a) Prepare environments for clinical procedures.	6, 11
(b) Maintain environments following clinical procedures.	6, 11

*U4 unit Contribute to the health, safety and security
of individuals and their equipment*

(c) Contribute to maintaining the safety and security of the environment.	5, 6
(d) Maintain personal standards of health, safety and security.	5, 6

*U5 unit Obtain, transmit and store information
relating to the delivery of a care service*

(a) Obtain information relating to care service delivery.	4
(b) Maintain, store and retrieve records.	4
(c) Receive and transmit information to others on request.	4

Index